Frontal Sinus Disease: Contemporary Management

Editors

JEAN ANDERSON ELOY
MICHAEL SETZEN

OTOLARYNGOLOGIC CLINICS OF NORTH AMERICA

www.oto.theclinics.com

August 2016 • Volume 49 • Number 4

ELSEVIER

1600 John F. Kennedy Boulevard ● Suite 1800 ● Philadelphia, Pennsylvania, 19103-2899

http://www.oto.theclinics.com

OTOLARYNGOLOGIC CLINICS OF NORTH AMERICA Volume 49, Number 4
August 2016 ISSN 0030-6665, ISBN-13: 978-0-323-44624-2

Editor: Jessica McCool
Developmental Editor: Alison Swety

Otolaryngologic Clinics of North America (ISSN 0030-6665) is published bimonthly by Elsevier, Inc., 360 Park Avenue South, New York, NY 10010-1710. Months of issue are February, April, June, August, October, and December. Business and Editorial Offices: 1600 John F. Kennedy Blvd., Suite 1800, Philadelphia, PA 19103-2899. Customer Service Office: 6277 Sea Harbor Drive, Orlando, FL 32887-4800. Periodicals postage paid at New York, NY and additional mailing offices. Subscription prices are $370.00 per year (US individuals), $765.00 per year (US institutions), $100.00 per year (US student/resident), $485.00 per year (Canadian individuals), $969.00 per year (Canadian institutions), $540.00 per year (international individuals), $969.00 per year (international institutions), $270.00 per year (international & Canadian student/resident). Foreign air speed delivery is included in all *Clinics'* subscription prices. All prices are subject to change without notice. **POSTMASTER:** Send address changes to *Otolaryngologic Clinics of North America*, Elsevier Health Sciences Division, Subscription Customer Service, 3251 Riverport Lane, Maryland Heights, MO 63043. **Telephone: 1-800-654-2452 (U.S. and Canada); 314-447-8871 (outside U.S. and Canada). Fax: 314-447-8029. E-mail: journalscustomerservice-usa@elsevier.com (for print support); journalsonlinesupport-usa@elsevier.com (for online support).**

Reprints. For copies of 100 or more of articles in this publication, please contact the Commercial Reprints Department, Elsevier Inc., 360 Park Avenue South, New York, NY 10010-1710. Tel.: 212-633-3874; Fax: 212-633-3820; E-mail: reprints@elsevier.com.

Otolaryngologic Clinics of North America is also published in Spanish by McGraw-Hill Interamericana Editores S.A., P.O. Box 5-237, 06500 Mexico D.F., Mexico.

Otolaryngologic Clinics of North America is covered in *MEDLINE/PubMed (Index Medicus), Current Contents/Clinical Medicine, Excerpta Medica, BIOSIS, Science Citation Index,* and *ISI/BIOMED.*

PROGRAM OBJECTIVE

The goal of the *Otolaryngologic Clinics of North America* is to provide information on the latest trends in patient management, the newest advances; and provide a sound basis for choosing treatment options in the field of otolaryngology.

LEARNING OBJECTIVES

Upon completion of this activity, participants will be able to:
1. Review the anatomy and pathology of the frontal sinus.
2. Discuss the evaluation and treatment of frontal sinusitis, including new approaches in surgical and medical management.
3. Recognize outcomes after frontal sinus surgery, and understand complication prevention.

ACCREDITATION

The Elsevier Office of Continuing Medical Education (EOCME) is accredited by the Accreditation Council for Continuing Medical Education (ACCME) to provide continuing medical education for physicians.

The EOCME designates this enduring material for a maximum of 15 *AMA PRA Category 1 Credit*(s)™. Physicians should claim only the credit commensurate with the extent of their participation in the activity.

All other health care professionals requesting continuing education credit for this enduring material will be issued a certificate of participation.

DISCLOSURE OF CONFLICTS OF INTEREST

The EOCME assesses conflict of interest with its instructors, faculty, planners, and other individuals who are in a position to control the content of CME activities. All relevant conflicts of interest that are identified are thoroughly vetted by EOCME for fair balance, scientific objectivity, and patient care recommendations. EOCME is committed to providing its learners with CME activities that promote improvements or quality in healthcare and not a specific proprietary business or a commercial interest.

The planning committee, staff, authors and editors listed below have identified no financial relationships or relationships to products or devices they or their spouse/life partner have with commercial interest related to the content of this CME activity:
Soly Baredes, MD, FACS; Henry P. Barham, MD; Adrianne Brigido; Roy R. Casiano, MD, FACS; Adam S. DeConde, MD; Dipan Desai, BS; Charles S. Ebert, MD, MPH; Jean Anderson Eloy, MD, FACS; Adam J. Folbe, MD; Anjali Fortna; Satish Govindaraj, MD; Yan Ho, MD; Elisa A. Illing, MD; Zeina R. Korban, MD; William Lawson, MD, DDS; Kristopher F. Lay, MD; James K. Liu, MD, FACS; Jessica McCool; Premkumar Nandhakumar; Gretchen M. Oakley, MD; Alok T. Saini, MD; Anne Morgan Selleck, MD; Michael Setzen, MD, FACS, FAAP; Susan Showalter; Michael J. Sillers, MD, FACS; Timothy L. Smith, MD, MPH; Maheep Sohal, MD; Megan Suermann; Peter F. Svider, MD; Bobby A. Tajudeen, MD; Brian D. Thorp, MD; Alejandro Vázquez, MD; Adam M. Zanation, MD.

The planning committee, staff, authors and editors listed below have identified financial relationships or relationships to products or devices they or their spouse/life partner have with commercial interest related to the content of this CME activity:
Nithin D. Adappa, MD is on the speakers' bureau for, and is a consultant/advisor for, Acclarent, Inc.
Seth M. Brown, MD, MBA is a consultant/advisor for Johnson & Johnson Services, Inc. and KARL STORZ GmbH & Co. KG.
Richard J. Harvey, MD, PhD is a consultant/advisor for Olympus America; Medtronic; Neilmed Pharmaceuticals, Inc; and Sequares; and has research support from Stallergenes Greer and ENT Technologies.
Belachew Tessema, MD is on the speakers' bureau for Intersent ENT, Inc and Acclarent, Inc, and is a consultant/advisor for Medtronic.
Bradford A. Woodworth, MD is a consultant/advisor for Smith & Nephew Inc; Cook Medical Inc; and Olympus America, and has research support from Cook Medical Inc.

UNAPPROVED/OFF-LABEL USE DISCLOSURE

The EOCME requires CME faculty to disclose to the participants:
1. When products or procedures being discussed are off-label, unlabelled, experimental, and/or investigational (not US Food and Drug Administration [FDA] approved); and
2. Any limitations on the information presented, such as data that are preliminary or that represent ongoing research, interim analyses, and/or unsupported opinions. Faculty may discuss information about pharmaceutical agents that is outside of FDA-approved labelling. This information is intended solely for CME

and is not intended to promote off-label use of these medications. If you have any questions, contact the medical affairs department of the manufacturer for the most recent prescribing information.

TO ENROLL
To enroll in the *Otolaryngologic Clinics of North America* Continuing Medical Education program, call customer service at 1-800-654-2452 or sign up online at http://www.theclinics.com/home/cme. The CME program is available to subscribers for an additional annual fee of USD 260.

METHOD OF PARTICIPATION
In order to claim credit, participants must complete the following:
1. Complete enrolment as indicated above.
2. Read the activity.
3. Complete the CME Test and Evaluation. Participants must achieve a score of 70% on the test. All CME Tests and Evaluations must be completed online.

CME INQUIRIES/SPECIAL NEEDS
For all CME inquiries or special needs, please contact elsevierCME@elsevier.com.

Contributors

EDITORS

JEAN ANDERSON ELOY, MD, FACS
Professor and Vice Chairman; Director, Rhinology and Sinus Surgery; Director, Otolaryngology Research; Co-Director, Endoscopic Skull Base Surgery Program, Department of Otolaryngology - Head and Neck Surgery, Center for Skull Base and Pituitary Surgery, Neurological Institute of New Jersey; Professor of Neurological Surgery, Professor of Ophthalmology and Visual Science, Departments of Neurological Surgery and Ophthalmology and Visual Science, Rutgers New Jersey Medical School, Newark, New Jersey

MICHAEL SETZEN, MD, FACS, FAAP
Past President, American Rhinologic Society (ARS); Past Chair Board of Governors, American Academy of Otolaryngology, Head and Neck Surgery (AAO-HNS); Chief Rhinology Section, North Shore University Hospital, Manhasset, New York; Clinical Associate Professor, Department of Otolaryngology, New York University School of Medicine; Adjunct Clinical Assistant Professor Otolaryngology, Weill Cornell University College of Medicine, New York, New York; Michael Setzen Otolaryngology, PC, Great Neck, New York

AUTHORS

NITHIN D. ADAPPA, MD
Department of Otorhinolaryngology - Head and Neck Surgery, The University of Pennsylvania, Philadelphia, Pennsylvania

SOLY BAREDES, MD, FACS
Center for Skull Base and Pituitary Surgery, Neurological Institute of New Jersey; Professor and Chair, Department of Otolaryngology - Head and Neck Surgery, Rutgers New Jersey Medical School, Newark, New Jersey

HENRY P. BARHAM, MD
Department of Otolaryngology - Head and Neck Surgery, Louisiana State University, New Orleans, Louisiana

SETH M. BROWN, MD, MBA
Division of Otolaryngology, Department of Surgery, University of Connecticut School of Medicine; The Connecticut Sinus Institute, Farmington, Connecticut

ROY R. CASIANO, MD, FACS
Professor and Vice Chairman; Rhinology Fellow; Department of Otolaryngology - Head and Neck Surgery, University of Miami, Miami, Florida

ADAM S. DeCONDE, MD
Assistant Professor of Rhinology and Skull Base Surgery, Division of Otolaryngology – Head and Neck Surgery, Department of Surgery, University of California, San Diego, San Diego, California

DIPAN DESAI, BS
Department of Otolaryngology - Head and Neck Surgery, University of North Carolina at Chapel Hill, Chapel Hill, North Carolina

CHARLES S. EBERT, MD, MPH
Associate Professor, Department of Otolaryngology - Head and Neck Surgery, University of North Carolina at Chapel Hill, Chapel Hill, North Carolina

JEAN ANDERSON ELOY, MD, FACS
Professor and Vice Chairman; Director, Rhinology and Sinus Surgery; Director, Otolaryngology Research; Co-Director, Endoscopic Skull Base Surgery Program, Department of Otolaryngology - Head and Neck Surgery, Center for Skull Base and Pituitary Surgery, Neurological Institute of New Jersey; Professor of Neurological Surgery, Professor of Ophthalmology and Visual Science, Departments of Neurological Surgery and Ophthalmology and Visual Science, Rutgers New Jersey Medical School, Newark, New Jersey

ADAM J. FOLBE, MD
Associate Professor; Director, Rhinology and Sinus Surgery, Department of Otolaryngology - Head and Neck Surgery; Department of Neurosurgery, Wayne State University School of Medicine, Detroit, Michigan

SATISH GOVINDARAJ, MD
Associate Professor, Otolaryngology - Head and Neck Surgery, Mount Sinai Medical Center, New York, New York

RICHARD J. HARVEY, MD, PhD
Rhinology and Skull Base Research Group, Applied Medical Research Centre, University of New South Wales; Faculty of Medicine and Health Sciences, Macquarie University, Sydney, Australia

YAN HO, MD
Icahn School of Medicine at Mount Sinai, New York, New York

ELISA A. ILLING, MD
Rhinology Fellow, Department of Otolaryngology, University of Alabama at Birmingham, Birmingham, Alabama

ZEINA R. KORBAN, MD
Rhinology Fellow, Department of Otolaryngology - Head and Neck Surgery, University of Miami, Miami, Florida

WILLIAM LAWSON, MD, DDS
Professor of Otolaryngology, Vice Chairman, Department of Otolaryngology - Head and Neck Surgery, Fellowship Director of Facial Plastic and Reconstructive Surgery, Icahn School of Medicine at Mount Sinai, New York, New York

KRISTOPHER F. LAY, MD
Alabama Nasal and Sinus Center, Birmingham, Alabama

JAMES K. LIU, MD, FACS
Associate Professor of Neurological Surgery and Otolaryngology - Head and Neck Surgery; Director, Center of Skull Base and Pituitary Surgery; Co-Director, Endoscopic Skull Base Surgery Program; Director, Surgical Neuro-Oncology and Brain Tumor Center, Departments of Neurological Surgery and Otolaryngology - Head and Neck Surgery, Neurological Institute of New Jersey, Rutgers New Jersey Medical School, Newark, New Jersey

GRETCHEN M. OAKLEY, MD
Rhinology and Skull Base Research Group, Applied Medical Research Centre, University of New South Wales, Sydney, Australia

ALOK T. SAINI, MD
Resident, Otolaryngology - Head and Neck Surgery, Mount Sinai Medical Center, New York, New York

ANNE MORGAN SELLECK, MD
Department of Otolaryngology - Head and Neck Surgery, University of North Carolina at Chapel Hill, Chapel Hill, North Carolina

MICHAEL SETZEN, MD, FACS, FAAP
Past President, American Rhinologic Society (ARS); Past Chair Board of Governors, American Academy of Otolaryngology, Head and Neck Surgery (AAO-HNS); Chief Rhinology Section, North Shore University Hospital, Manhasset, New York; Clinical Associate Professor, Department of Otolaryngology, New York University School of Medicine; Adjunct Clinical Assistant Professor Otolaryngology, Weill Cornell University College of Medicine, New York, New York; Michael Setzen Otolaryngology, PC, Great Neck, New York

MICHAEL J. SILLERS, MD, FACS
Alabama Nasal and Sinus Center; Clinical Professor, Otolaryngology - Head and Neck Surgery, The University of Alabama-Birmingham, Birmingham, Alabama

TIMOTHY L. SMITH, MD, MPH
Professor of Rhinology and Skull Base Surgery, Division of Rhinology, Sinus, and Skull Base Surgery, Department of Otolaryngology - Head and Neck Surgery, Oregon Sinus Center, Oregon Health and Science University, Portland, Oregon

MAHEEP SOHAL, MD
Division of Otolaryngology, Department of Surgery, University of Connecticut School of Medicine, Farmington, Connecticut

PETER F. SVIDER, MD
Otolaryngology Resident, Department of Otolaryngology - Head and Neck Surgery, Wayne State University School of Medicine, Detroit, Michigan

BOBBY A. TAJUDEEN, MD
Department of Otorhinolaryngology - Head and Neck Surgery, The University of Pennsylvania, Philadelphia, Pennsylvania

BELACHEW TESSEMA, MD
Division of Otolaryngology, Department of Surgery, University of Connecticut School of Medicine; The Connecticut Sinus Institute, Farmington, Connecticut

BRIAN D. THORP, MD
Assistant Professor, Department of Otolaryngology - Head and Neck Surgery, University of North Carolina at Chapel Hill, Chapel Hill, North Carolina

ALEJANDRO VÁZQUEZ, MD
Fellow in Rhinology, Sinus, and Endoscopic Skull Base Surgery, Department of Otolaryngology - Head and Neck Surgery, Neurological Institute of New Jersey, Rutgers New Jersey Medical School, Newark, New Jersey

BRADFORD A. WOODWORTH, MD
James J. Hicks Professor of Otolaryngology and Residency Program Director, Associate Scientist at the Gregory Fleming James Cystic Fibrosis Research Center, Department of Otolaryngology, University of Alabama at Birmingham, Birmingham, Alabama

ADAM M. ZANATION, MD
Associate Professor, Departments of Otolaryngology - Head and Neck Surgery and Neurosurgery, University of North Carolina at Chapel Hill, Chapel Hill, North Carolina

Contents

The frontal sinus is the most complex of all paranasal sinuses. Given its proximity to the cranial vault and orbit, frontal sinus pathology can progress to involve these structures and lead to significant morbidity, or even mortality. Surgical management of the frontal sinus is technically challenging. Various open and endoscopic surgical techniques are available to the otolaryngologist. This article presents an overview of the major disease entities that affect the frontal sinus, with a special emphasis on treatment principles and surgical management.

Management of frontal sinusitis can be challenging for even the most experienced otolaryngologists. A thorough understanding of the anatomy and pathophysiology of the frontal sinus is essential to properly manage disease affecting the frontal sinus. Being able to distinguish acute viral from acute bacterial and acute from chronic sinusitis is crucial because these distinctions guide appropriate management. Nasal endoscopy can confirm diagnosis, and radiologic imaging, including computed tomography and MRI, is often a necessary adjunct that aids in determining appropriate therapeutic decisions. One must be aware of the many procedures used in the surgical treatment of frontal sinusitis.

Rhinosinusitis is a term that has long been used to describe a diverse disease entity that encompasses several related but distinct conditions involving the paranasal sinuses. Frontal sinusitis represents one such entity with its own unique treatment considerations. Like rhinosinusitis as a whole, the role of medical management in the treatment of frontal sinusitis cannot be overlooked. Contemporary medical management of frontal sinusitis requires recognition of the unique disease process with implementation of targeted therapies aimed at addressing the specific pathophysiology.

Comprehension of the complex anatomic variants comprising the frontal sinus outflow tract is essential for successful surgical intervention.

Deviation from sound technique increases the potential for a variety of deleterious sequelae, including recurrent disease as well as catastrophic intracranial and orbital injury. Furthermore, incomplete removal of elements occluding the frontal recess can result in severe stenosis that can increase the difficulty of further interventions. This review covers anatomic considerations that should be kept in mind when performing frontal sinus surgery.

Frontal recess dissection proposes many challenges to the surgeon. These challenges stem from its highly variable nature, small caliber, difficult visualization, and proximity to vital structures such as the skull base and orbit. As such, delicate mucosal-sparing dissection of the frontal recess with proper instrumentation is paramount to minimize scar formation and ensure patency. Here, the article explores key instrumentation in frontal recess surgery with an emphasis on hand instruments and adjunctive technologies.

This review covers potential complications of frontal sinus surgical management and strategies for prevention of these complications. Accordingly, recent advances in frontal sinus surgical techniques are described, and the management of complications stemming both from these and traditional techniques are detailed.

The decision to operate on the frontal sinus is based on persistent symptoms that have been refractory to appropriate medical therapy with associated radiographic evidence of disease by computed tomography. There is currently no evidence to support operating on radiographically negative frontal sinuses, regardless of the availability of technology or site of service options. There are many surgical procedures as well as a variety of different technologies available for the treatment of symptomatic, medically refractory frontal sinus disease. Balloon catheter dilation can be performed safely in an office setting with outcomes comparable to those in traditional operating room settings.

The frontal sinus can present a challenging surgical dissection for the endoscopic surgeon. Image guidance as a surgical adjunct has become widely accepted for surgeries in this area. It can help verify vital structures and manage disorienting surgical conditions, improving surgeon confidence in performing safer and more complete surgery. It is relied upon heavily for placement of limited external frontal sinusotomies for disease beyond the endoscopic reach, and for mapping the frontal sinus for osteoplastic flap bony cuts. Its use has contributed to the expanding role of endoscopic surgical approaches for paranasal sinus inflammatory and neoplastic disease.

 Video content accompanies this article at http://www.oto. theclinics.com.

The mainstay of frontal sinus surgery for chronic rhinosinusitis is to achieve and maintain an adequate frontal outflow tract. Using a stepwise approach and identifying critical endoscopic anatomic landmarks, to minimize complications and obtain long-term good endoscopic surgical results, should achieve this. The goal is to relieve the patient's symptoms, restore functional mucociliary flow, achieve a wide frontal sinus ostium, and prevent long-term scarring and stenosis. Meticulous dissection and appropriate use of instrumentation and techniques aids in preventing unnecessary damage to normal mucosa while achieving one's goal of an adequate surgical ostium.

 Video content accompanies this article at http://www.oto. theclinics.com.

Frontal sinus surgery has long been technically challenging in terms of access and chronic disease management. Decades of experience and advances in technology have led to the widespread use of various surgical approaches to the frontal sinus. Modifications to these existing procedures have been described to minimize unnecessarily invasive approaches. The lack of a classification that incorporates the newly described modifications prompts the proposal of a new classification. Eloy I–III incorporates all the previously described approaches as well as 3 recently published, and 1 newly described, procedures.

Endoscopic sinus surgery is an effective intervention at improving quality of life for patients with medically refractory chronic rhinosinusitis. The evidence supporting frontal sinusotomy is limited to single institution case series. However, the data for Draf IIa frontal sinusotomy do demonstrate that most patients experience lasting frontal sinus patency on postoperative endoscopic examination and improvements in quality of life. Salvage endoscopic frontal sinus surgery via a Draf III shows high rates of neo-ostium patency and subjective improvements in symptoms at a 2-year time point in case series.

OTOLARYNGOLOGIC CLINICS
OF NORTH AMERICA

RELATED INTEREST

Neuroimaging Clinics of North America
November 2015 (Vol. 25, Issue 4)
Imaging of Paranasal Sinuses
Varsha M. Joshi, *Editor*
Available at: http://www.neuroimaging.theclinics.com/

THE CLINICS ARE AVAILABLE ONLINE!
Access your subscription at:
www.theclinics.com

Preface

Frontal Sinus Disease: Contemporary Management

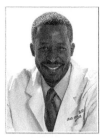
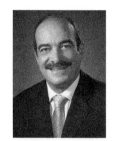

Jean Anderson Eloy, MD, FACS   Michael Setzen, MD, FACS, FAAP
Editors

Rhinosinusitis affects an estimated 1 in 7 adults in the United States. Otolaryngologists are intimately involved in the care of patients with rhinosinusitis and other upper airway inflammatory conditions through medical management and procedures such as endoscopic sinus surgery. The frontal sinus is considered the most difficult of the paranasal sinuses to manage. Frontal sinusitis is typically treated medically, with surgical interventions reserved for the most recalcitrant cases. Both private practitioners and academic physicians manage frontal sinusitis. Over the last two decades, new advances in medical management, newer understanding of the sinonasal anatomy, improved surgical instrumentation and optical devices, and newer surgical techniques to approach the frontal sinus have brought significant changes in the understanding and overall management of frontal sinus disease.

In this issue of *Otolaryngologic Clinics of North America* devoted to frontal sinus disease, we have attempted to present and discuss a comprehensive approach to the management of frontal sinus disease. We consider it a great honor to guest-edit this important issue on "Frontal Sinus Disease: Contemporary Management" and

Michael Setzen: Speaker's Bureau for Meda and Advisory Board for Merck and Lannett (not related to the current subject).

Otolaryngol Clin N Am 49 (2016) xv–xvi
http://dx.doi.org/10.1016/j.otc.2016.05.017   **oto.theclinics.com**

hope that this issue will be valuable to otolaryngologists managing a variety of frontal sinus pathologies.

Jean Anderson Eloy, MD, FACS
Department of Otolaryngology - Head and Neck Surgery
Center for Skull Base and Pituitary Surgery
Neurological Institute of New Jersey
Department of Neurological Surgery
Department of Ophthalmology
and Visual Science
Rutgers New Jersey Medical School
90 Bergen Street, Suite 8100
Newark, NJ 07103, USA

Michael Setzen, MD, FACS, FAAP
Chief Rhinology Section
North Shore University Hospital
Manhasset, NY 11030, USA

Department of Otolaryngology
New York University School of Medicine
New York, NY 10016, USA

Michael Setzen Otolaryngology, PC
600 Northern Boulevard, Suite 312
Great Neck, NY 11021, USA

E-mail addresses:
jean.anderson.eloy@gmail.com (J.A. Eloy)
michaelsetzen@gmail.com (M. Setzen)

Overview of Frontal Sinus Pathology and Management

Alejandro Vázquez, MD[a], Soly Baredes, MD[a,b],
Michael Setzen, MD[c,d], Jean Anderson Eloy, MD[a,b,e,f,g],*

KEYWORDS

- Frontal sinus • Frontal recess • Frontal sinus drainage pathway
- Endoscopic sinus surgery • Draf classification • Modified Lothrop procedure
- Chronic rhinosinusitis • Complications of rhinosinusitis

KEY POINTS

- The frontal sinus is the most anatomically complex of the paranasal sinuses and subject to a great degree of anatomic variations, enough variations, in fact, that they can be used to distinguish 1 monozygotic twin from the other.
- When surgery is indicated, the approach of choice is usually endoscopic. However, even in the age of modern endoscopy and stereotactic image guidance, endoscopic frontal sinus surgery is challenging.
- Recent advances in frontal sinus management include the use of intraoperative stereotactic image guidance, as well as the availability of minimally invasive office-based balloon catheter dilation procedures.

Financial Disclosures: None.
Conflicts of Interest: Speaker's Bureau for Meda and Advisory Board for Merck and Lannett (not related to current subject) (M. Setzen).
[a] Department of Otolaryngology–Head and Neck Surgery, Rutgers New Jersey Medical School, Newark, NJ, USA; [b] Center for Skull Base and Pituitary Surgery, Neurological Institute of New Jersey, Rutgers New Jersey Medical School, Newark, NJ, USA; [c] Rhinology Section, North Shore University Hospital, Manhasset, NY, USA; [d] Department of Otolaryngology, New York University School of Medicine, New York, NY, USA; [e] Department of Neurological Surgery, Rutgers New Jersey Medical School, Newark, NJ, USA; [f] Department of Ophthalmology and Visual Science, Rutgers New Jersey Medical School, Newark, NJ, USA; [g] Endoscopic Skull Base Surgery Program, Department of Otolaryngology–Head and Neck Surgery, Neurological Institute of New Jersey, Rutgers New Jersey Medical School, 90 Bergen Street, Suite 8100, Newark, NJ 07103, USA
* Corresponding author. Endoscopic Skull Base Surgery Program, Department of Otolaryngology–Head and Neck Surgery, Neurological Institute of New Jersey, Rutgers New Jersey Medical School, 90 Bergen Street, Suite 8100, Newark, NJ 07103.
E-mail address: jean.anderson.eloy@gmail.com

INTRODUCTION

The frontal sinuses are the most complex of all paranasal sinuses. Their intrinsic variability and their anatomic location have historically made it difficult to access them surgically. Even today, despite the existence of sophisticated endoscopy systems, specialized instrumentation, and stereotactic navigation, the frontal sinuses still command a great deal of respect. This article presents an overview of frontal sinus anatomy, pathology, and principles of management for the major pathologic entities affecting them.

ANATOMY OF THE FRONTAL SINUS

The frontal sinuses are absent at birth; they are visible radiographically as early as age 4. Paralleling general craniofacial growth, frontal sinus expansion peaks during adolescence and stops by around age 19. Unilateral or bilateral aplasia is seen in about 5% of people.[1]

Frontal sinus anatomy is highly variable: in fact, it is unique to each individual, such that even monozygotic twins can be distinguished from each another on the basis of their frontal sinus configuration alone.[2] Indeed, frontal sinus anatomy is regarded as a reliable means of personal identification in the forensic sciences.[3]

The frontal sinuses are paired asymmetric structures separated by a bony septum (the intersinus septum). The greater part of their volume lies within the anterior aspect of the frontal bone and is bounded by anterior and posterior tables. Patients with marked pneumatization may have a pronounced lateral recess, which can be difficult to reach endoscopically. Inferiorly, each sinus narrows into an obliquely oriented transition point known as the frontal ostium, which, in the sagittal plane, is bounded by the nasofrontal buttress (also referred to as nasal or frontal beak) anteriorly and by the skull base posteriorly. The frontal ostium marks the superior limit of what is known as the frontal recess. Although this term is in common usage, it is somewhat imprecise and difficult to define anatomically, and some have argued for a more inclusive and accurate alternative, the frontal sinus drainage pathway (FSDP).[4]

The FSDP can be divided into superior and inferior compartments. The superior compartment lies between the anteroinferior frontal bone and the anterosuperior ethmoid bone (ie, slightly above the agger nasi cell and ethmoid bulla), and it may or may not contain air cells. The inferior compartment is either the ethmoid infundibulum (if the uncinate process attaches to the skull base) or the middle meatus (if the uncinate attaches to the medial orbital wall).[4] A variety of anatomic structures and factors can influence the patency of either compartment; these include: agger nasi cell (presence and degree of pneumatization); supraorbital ethmoid cells; frontal cells (types 1 through 4); suprabullar cells; and interfrontal sinus septal cells (**Fig. 1**). Surgical anatomy is reviewed in greater detail by Folbe AJ, Svider PF, Eloy JA: Anatomic Considerations in Frontal Sinus Surgery, later in this issue.

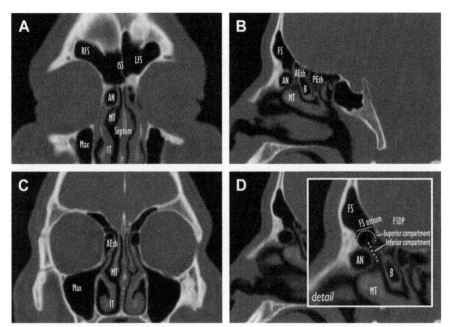

Fig. 1. Coronal (*A, C*) and sagittal (*B, D*) CT scan depicting the anatomy of the frontal sinus drainage pathway and surrounding structures. AEth, anterior ethmoid cells; AN, agger nasi cell; B, ethmoid bulla; FS, frontal sinus; FSDP, frontal sinus drainage pathway; ISS, intersinus septum; IT, inferior turbinate; LFS, left frontal sinus; Max, maxillary sinus; MT, middle turbinate; PEth, posterior ethmoid cells; RFS, right frontal sinus.

OVERVIEW OF FRONTAL SINUS PATHOLOGY AND MANAGEMENT

This section presents a brief overview of the main pathologic processes that affect the frontal sinus, with an emphasis on management principles. Most of these entities affect the frontal sinuses less commonly than the remainder of the sinonasal tract; in such cases, the topics are discussed broadly, since pathophysiology, workup, and management do not differ much.

Acute Rhinosinusitis

Acute rhinosinusitis is defined clinically as the presence of up to 4 weeks of purulent rhinorrhea accompanied by either nasal obstruction, facial pain/pressure/fullness, or both. In the early phase of the disease, the etiology is presumed to be viral; however, if there is failure to improve within 10 days, or if there is worsening of symptoms after an initial improvement, then a diagnosis of acute bacterial rhinosinusitis (ABRS) is made.[5] Acute frontal sinusitis is considerably less common than sinusitis of the maxillary and ethmoid sinuses; however, it is difficult to evaluate this given that radiographic imaging is not routinely indicated in the management of this disorder. Frontal sinus involvement is most common in adolescent boys and young men, presumably due to the peak vascularity and development, which occurs between ages 7 and 20 years; the reason for the apparent gender predilection remains unclear.

The treatment of uncomplicated ABRS (defined as ABRS without evidence of extension outside of the sinonasal tract) is pharmacologic. Initial antibiotic selection is empiric, aimed at covering the most common bacterial pathogens, namely, *Streptococcus pneumoniae*, *Hemophilus influenzae*, and *Moraxella catarrhalis*.[5] Complicated ABRS is often polymicrobial in etiology. Treatment is with broad-spectrum intravenous antibiotic therapy and often surgical intervention to address the complication and/or the sinonasal tract pathology. Recently, the *Streptococcus anginosus* group (also known as the *S milleri* group or group F streptococci) has emerged as an important group of pathogens responsible for severe suppurative complications of rhinosinusitis. In one study, *S milleri* was isolated in 67% of cases of sinogenic intracranial abscess in children.[6,7] Medical management of ABRS is discussed in further detail by Sohal M, Tessema B, Brown SM: Medical Management of Frontal Sinusitis, later in this issue.

CHRONIC RHINOSINUSITIS

Chronic rhinosinusitis (CRS) is defined as inflammation of the sinonasal tract lasting more than 12 weeks.[5] Although this definition has a certain practical utility, it fails to capture the complexity of CRS. Most forms of CRS fall into one of two categories: CRS with polyposis or CRS without polyposis. However, CRS may also represent a common endpoint for a variety of systemic disorders.[8] In discussions of CRS management, the concept of maximal medical therapy is often cited as the threshold beyond which surgical management is indicated, but a universal definition of this concept does not exist. In a 2007 survey of 388 American Rhinologic Society members, Dubin and colleagues[9] found that oral antibiotics (a 3–4-week course) and nasal steroids were the only 2 modalities that greater than 90% of respondents considered part of their standard regimens. Oral steroids, saline irrigation, and allergy testing were employed less consistently (50%–90%).

Clinical and radiographic assessments after completion of medical therapy determine the persistence or resolution of paranasal sinus disease. Just as with all sinonasal disease, high-resolution computed tomography (CT) is essential to the evaluation of frontal sinus disease. CT may serve a diagnostic purpose in revealing unfavorable FSDP or frontal sinus anatomy, and it also serves as a roadmap. In some cases, frontal sinus disease may be attributable to outflow pathway obstruction at the level of the anterior ethmoid sinuses, and management of the anterior ethmoid air cells can be sufficient. In other cases, cannulations of the FSDP and balloon dilation are sufficient to manage limited disease. However, in many cases, surgical management of the frontal sinuses requires a formal frontal sinusotomy or a more extended dissection (such as a Draf III procedure). Evaluation and decision making are discussed in greater detail by Saini AT and Govindaraj S: Evaluation and Decision Making in Frontal Sinus Surgery, in this issue; medical management is reviewed by Sohal M, Tessema B, Brown SM: Medical Management of Frontal Sinusitis, later in this issue.

Complications of Frontal Sinusitis

Complications of rhinosinusitis are uncommon, occurring in only 1% to 3% of all cases. In the preantibiotic era, postseptal orbital complications were associated with a high incidence of vision loss (as high as 20%) and intracranial complications with high rates of mortality (up to 17%).[10]

Orbital complications of rhinosinusitis may arise by direct extension or via retrograde thrombophlebitis. Several modifications have been made to the original classification scheme proposed by Chandler and colleagues in 1970. In spite of key differences, they share at least 2 common features: preseptal involvement represents the least severe of the complications, and cavernous sinus thrombosis (CST) represents the most severe. In the Groote Schuur Hospital classification, CST is considered an intracranial complication. The rest are organized thus, in approximate order of severity:

1. Preseptal disease (either cellulitis or, less commonly, eyelid abscess)
2. Postseptal extraconal involvement (either subperiosteal phlegmon/cellulitis or abscess) (**Fig. 2**)
3. Postseptal intraconal involvement (either cellulitis or abscess)
4. Orbital abscess (either localized or diffuse)[11]

Preseptal cellulitis generally responds quickly to systemic broad-spectrum antibiotics. Theoretically, a diagnosis of preseptal cellulitis can be made on purely clinical grounds, therefore obviating the need for CT scanning; however, in practice, it is common to obtain CT scans with any suspected orbital complication, and patients will often have had imaging by the time ophthalmologic consultation is requested. Surgical therapy in preseptal cellulitis is considered only in cases of antibiotic failure or overt disease progression.

By contrast, postseptal complications often require surgical intervention. Surgical indications include abscess formation, signs of severe orbital disease (eg, vision loss or ophthalmoplegia), and failure to respond to appropriate antibiotic therapy. When indicated, surgery should address orbital and sinonasal disease simultaneously.[12,13] Depending on the specific complication, orbital disease may be approached via open orbitotomy, or, in some cases, via a transnasal endoscopic approach (eg, in the case of a medially located subperiosteal abscess). Historically, sinonasal disease was approached via external frontoethmoidectomy or frontal sinus trephination. The treatment of choice today is endoscopic sinus surgery (ESS). However, it should be noted that acute sinonasal inflammation may make endoscopic frontal sinus surgery quite difficult, and open techniques remain an option.[14]

Intracranial complications of rhinosinusitis can lead to severe morbidity or even death. These include meningitis, epidural abscess, subdural empyema (**Fig. 3**), brain abscess, cavernous sinus thrombosis, superior sagittal sinus thrombosis, and frontal bone osteomyelitis. In a patient with rhinosinusitis, the presence of fever and acute or progressive headache may herald the onset of an intracranial complication; however, in some cases, it may not be clinically evident until more severe symptoms (such as neurologic deficits or changes in mental status) arise. In addition to broad-spectrum

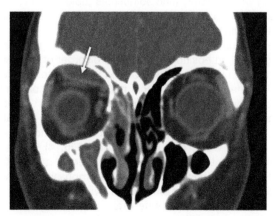

Fig. 2. Contrast-enhanced coronal CT showing a right-sided acute bacterial rhinosinusitis (frontal, ethmoid and maxillary) complicated by an orbital subperiosteal abscess (*arrow*).

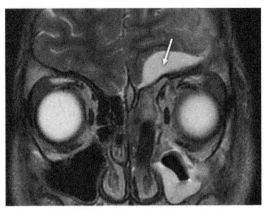

Fig. 3. T2-weighted coronal MRI showing a left subdural empyema (*arrow*) in a patient with acute bacterial rhinosinusitis (frontal, ethmoid and maxillary).

antibiotics, management of intracranial complications usually involves surgical intervention. The sinonasal infection and intracranial complication should be addressed simultaneously.[13,15] Ideally, sinonasal surgery should clear all infectious material from the frontal sinus and establish adequate/safe outflow. However, given a choice between the 2 goals, priority should be given to drainage; hence, trephination remains a viable temporizing option if formal frontal sinusotomy is not feasible.

Fungal Rhinosinusitis

Fungal disorders of the sinonasal tract fall into one of two categories: invasive and noninvasive.[16] Acute invasive fungal rhinosinusitis (AIFRS) is a fulminant, life-threatening, necrotizing infection that most commonly affects immunocompromised patients. The frontal sinus is the least common site of involvement (4.8% of cases in 1 series, and always in conjunction with other sinuses).[17] CT findings are generally nonspecific, with thickening of the sinonasal mucosa as the most consistent finding. MRI may help in characterizing the extent of extranasal disease. Treatment consists of endoscopic surgical debridement of all necrotic tissue until healthy, bleeding tissue is uncovered, along with systemic (and sometimes topical) antifungal therapy. Given the dismal survival rates of patients with AIFRS, extensive or radical surgical resection should be weighed carefully.[18]

Allergic fungal rhinosinusitis (AFRS) is the sinonasal analogue of allergic bronchopulmonary aspergillosis, an eosinophil-mediated disorder of the lower airways. It is characterized by typical histopathologic features that include the presence of eosinophils and fungal elements within a mucin matrix. AFRS is primarily a disorder of local immune dysfunction rather than an infectious process.[8] Clinically, it presents with sinonasal polyposis, usually in atopic patients. The frontal sinus may be involved in up to 71% of cases. Characteristic CT findings include sinus expansion, remodeling of the sinus walls, and bony erosion (**Fig. 4**).[19] These changes are thought to develop from the sequestration of allergic mucin. Surgery is often required in AFRS, and 2 principles should be emphasized: first, the complete removal of allergic mucin and diseased tissue (while preserving healthy mucosa); and second, the establishment of a safe drainage pathway that provides access for adjunctive topical therapy. The importance of postoperative maintenance therapy cannot be overemphasized.[20]

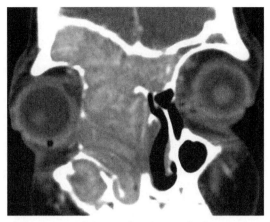

Fig. 4. Coronal CT of the paranasal sinuses showing marked expansion of the right frontal sinus, frontal sinus recess, and ethmoid sinus by allergic mucin (note the heterogenous appearance).

Benign Lesions of the Frontal Sinus

Mucoceles are mucus-filled cystic lesions lined with respiratory epithelium. Although histologically benign, they are expansile and have the capacity to erode bone (**Fig. 5**). This process is partly mechanical and partly biochemical; cytokines produced as part

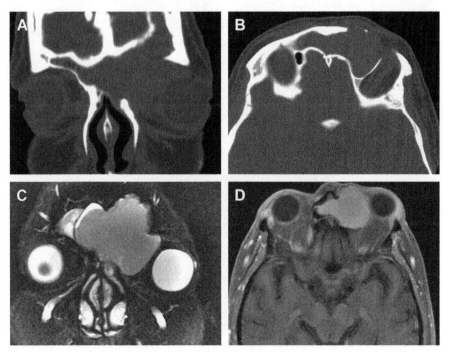

Fig. 5. Coronal (*A*) and axial (*B*) CT of a large left-sided frontal sinus mucocele with marked displacement of the left globe. T2-weighted coronal MRI (*C*) and T1-weighted axial MRI (*D*) of the same patient showing the large mucocele.

of a local immune response promote bone resorption and remodeling.[21] Traditionally, treatment of frontal sinus mucoceles entailed open surgery, often with sinus obliteration.[22] With the advent of sinonasal endoscopy and advanced frontal sinus operative techniques (ie, Draf IIb/III, discussed later), the trend shifted toward endoscopic marsupialization. This has proven to be an effective method of managing even very large or very lateral lesions.[23]

The entity known as Pott's puffy tumor (**Fig. 6**) is not, as the name would suggest, a neoplasm; rather, it is a subperiosteal abscess of the frontal bone associated with a severe underlying infection of the frontal sinus. Spread of infection into the subperiosteal space occurs either by thrombophlebitis or direct extension through osteomyelitic bone. The typical clinical appearance, which gives its name, is that of a doughy/pitting swelling of the forehead. Associated symptoms include fever, rhinorrhea, pain, and fever.[24]

Several other benign lesions can affect the frontal sinuses, including osteoma (**Fig. 7**A) (and other fibro-osseous lesions, such as fibrous dysplasia [**Fig. 7**B] and ossifying fibroma [**Fig. 7**C]) and inverted papilloma (IP). Osteomas are managed surgically, either by ESS, open, or combined approaches. IP is a premalignant lesion, with an approximate rate of malignant conversion of 10% to 15%. It arises most commonly from the lateral nasal wall, where the treatment of choice is medial maxillectomy (usually in the form of an endoscopic modified medial maxillectomy). The 2 fundamental principles of IP management are gross total resection and the creation of a cavity amenable to full visualization for in-office surveillance. Frontal sinus IP is considerably

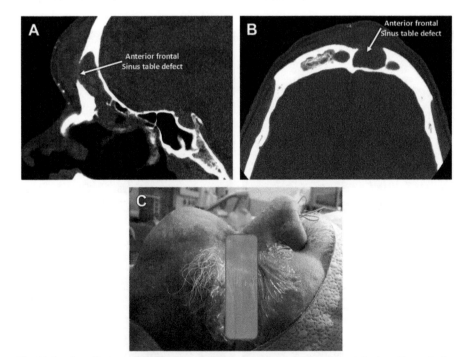

Fig. 6. Pott's puffy tumor. (*A*) Sagittal and (*B*) axial CT showing a bony defect on the anterior table of the frontal sinus, with opacification of the sinus and prominent soft tissue swelling with subcutaneous forehead collection. (*C*) Photograph showing characteristic clinical appearance.

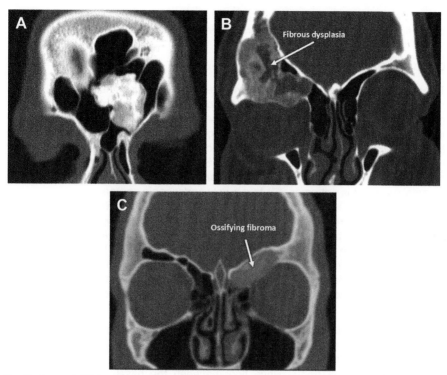

Fig. 7. Coronal CT showing various fibro-osseous lesions of the frontal sinus: (*A*) osteoma, (*B*) fibrous dysplasia, and (*C*) ossifying fibroma.

less common, but the same principles can be extrapolated. A recent systematic review of frontal sinus IP showed a recurrence rate of 22.4% (for a combination of open surgery and ESS).[25]

Malignant Neoplasms of the Frontal Sinus

Frontal sinus malignancy is rare, comprising less than 2% of all cases of sinonasal malignancy (which in turn make up only about 3% of all head and neck malignancies).[26] Most sinonasal tumors are epithelial in origin, with squamous cell carcinoma overwhelmingly more common than any other histology. The management of frontal sinus malignancy is discussed by Desai D, Selleck AM, Thorp B, et al: Management of Frontal Sinus Tumors, later in this issue.

Disorders of Skull Base Integrity—Cerebrospinal Fluid Leak and Encephaloceles

Most cerebrospinal fluid (CSF) leaks are either spontaneous or post-traumatic. In the latter case, there is usually an obvious history of head trauma that involves the posterior table or FSDP; in the former, patients tend to be obese, middle-aged women (often with undiagnosed intracranial hypertension). Repair of CSF leaks (see Illing EA, Woodworth BA: Management of Frontal Sinus Cerebrospinal Fluid Leaks and Encephaloceles, in this issue) may be carried out via ESS, open surgery, or combined approaches, and with a variety of different graft materials, depending on location and extent of the defect. When associated with encephaloceles, these are resected and/or obliterated with bipolar electrocautery prior to repair of the skull base defect. Intrathecal fluorescein aids in the intraoperative detection of the defect.[27]

OVERVIEW OF FRONTAL SINUS SURGERY

The history of frontal sinus surgery is long; trephination of the sinus appears to have been performed as early as the mid-18th century. External frontoethmoidectomy and various radical procedures were first performed in the late 19th century, and the well-known Lothrop procedure was described in 1914.[28] The advent of ESS in the early 1980s has obviated the need for most open surgery; however, these techniques (see Lawson W, Ho Y: Open Frontal Sinus Surgery: A Lost Art, in this issue) remain a valuable part of the rhinologist's armamentarium, since there will always be pathology that is not amenable to a purely endoscopic approach.

Because of its anatomic position, the frontal sinus is the most difficult to approach endoscopically. It requires a thorough understanding of complex 3-dimensional anatomy, the ability to maintain spatial orientation while using 30° and 70° angled telescopes, and precise control of angled instrumentation, including high-speed drills. In 1991, Wolfgang Draf introduced a classification scheme for endoscopic frontal sinus surgery that has stood the test of time (see Korban ZR, Casiano RR: Standard Endoscopic Approaches in Frontal Sinus Surgery: Technical Pearls and Approach Selection, in this issue). It can be summarized as follows:

I: anterior ethmoidectomy, without direct instrumentation of the FSDP

IIA: simple frontal sinusotomy (removal of anterior ethmoid and frontal cells protruding into the FSDP)

IIB: removal of the frontal sinus floor between the nasal septum and lamina papiracea

III: (modified Lothrop procedure): creation of a common cavity with median drainage

Several modifications to these approaches have been described by Eloy and colleagues in previous reports (see Eloy JA, Vazquez A, Liu JK, et al: Endoscopic Approaches to the Frontal Sinus: Modifications of the Existing Techniques and Proposed Classification, in this issue). A class IIC approach, or modified hemi-Lothrop procedure, provides enhanced access to the lateral recess and supraorbital cells[29–32]; a class IID approach, or modified mini-Lothrop procedure, provides contralateral drainage of a diseased frontal sinus when the ipsilateral approach is not feasible.[33,34] A class IIE approach, or modified subtotal-Lothrop procedure, establishes bilateral drainage and provides bilateral frontal sinus access but preserves some degree of native anatomy by keeping intact one of the frontal sinus recesses.[35,36]

Advanced frontal sinus surgery has been facilitated in recent years by stereotactic intraoperative navigation technology (see Oakley GM, Barham HP, Harvey RJ: Utility of Image-Guidance in Frontal Sinus Surgery, in this issue). In some cases, even the most conservative surgical approaches have been obviated by minimally invasive balloon–dilation techniques (see Sillers MJ, Lay KF: Balloon Catheter Dilation of the Frontal Sinus Ostium, in this issue).

SUMMARY

Management of frontal sinus pathology in general remains among the more challenging subjects in otolaryngology, and frontal sinus surgery specifically represents one of the most interesting facets of surgical rhinologic practice. This issue aims to present a detailed, up-to-date, evidenced-based review of the issues most relevant to frontal sinus management today.

REFERENCES

1. Fatu C, Puisoru M, Rotaru M, et al. Morphometric evaluation of the frontal sinus in relation to age. Ann Anat 2006;188:275–80.
2. Kjaer I, Pallisgaard C, Brock-Jacobsen MT. Frontal sinus dimensions can differ significantly between individuals within a monozygotic twin pair, indicating environmental influence on sinus sizes. Acta Otolaryngol 2012;132:988–94.
3. Besana JL, Rogers TL. Personal identification using the frontal sinus. J Forensic Sci 2010;55:584–9.
4. Daniels DL, Mafee MF, Smith MM, et al. The frontal sinus drainage pathway and related structures. AJNR Am J Neuroradiol 2003;24:1618–27.
5. Rosenfeld RM, Piccirillo JF, Chandrasekhar SS, et al. Clinical practice guideline (update): adult sinusitis. Otolaryngol Head Neck Surg 2015;152:S1–39.
6. Patel AP, Masterson L, Deutsch CJ, et al. Management and outcomes in children with sinogenic intracranial abscesses. Int J Pediatr Otorhinolaryngol 2015;79: 868–73.
7. Olwoch IP. Microbiology of acute complicated bacterial sinusitis at the University of the Witwatersrand. S Afr Med J 2010;100:529–33.
8. Carniol ET, Svider PF, Vazquez AV, et al. Epidemiology and pathophysiology of chronic rhinosinusitis. In: Batra PS, Han JK, editors. Practical medical and surgical management of chronic rhinosinusitis. New York: Springer International Publishing; 2015. p. 3–18.
9. Dubin MG, Liu C, Lin SY, et al. American Rhinologic Society member survey on "maximal medical therapy" for chronic rhinosinusitis. Am J Rhinol 2007;21:483–8.
10. Osguthorpe JD, Hochman M. Inflammatory sinus diseases affecting the orbit. Otolaryngol Clin North Am 1993;26:657–71.
11. Mortimore S, Wormald PJ. The Groote Schuur hospital classification of the orbital complications of sinusitis. J Laryngol Otol 1997;111:719–23.
12. Ozkurt FE, Ozkurt ZG, Gul A, et al. Managment of orbital complications of sinusitis. Arq Bras Oftalmol 2014;77:293–6.
13. Adelson R, Marple B. Orbital complications of frontal sinusitis. In: Kountakis S, Senior B, Draf W, editors. The frontal sinus. Heidelberg (Germany): Springer Berlin; 2005. p. 59–66.
14. Teinzer F, Stammberger H, Tomazic PV. Transnasal endoscopic treatment of orbital complications of acute sinusitis: the graz concept. Ann Otol Rhinol Laryngol 2015;124:368–73.
15. McIntosh DL, Mahadevan M. Frontal sinus mini-trephination for acute sinusitis complicated by intracranial infection. Int J Pediatr Otorhinolaryngol 2007;71: 1573–7.
16. Ferguson BJ. Definitions of fungal rhinosinusitis. Otolaryngol Clin North Am 2000; 33:227–35.
17. Gillespie MB, O'Malley BW Jr, Francis HW. An approach to fulminant invasive fungal rhinosinusitis in the immunocompromised host. Arch Otolaryngol Head Neck Surg 1998;124:520–6.
18. Monroe MM, McLean M, Sautter N, et al. Invasive fungal rhinosinusitis: a 15-year experience with 29 patients. Laryngoscope 2013;123:1583–7.
19. Mukherji SK, Figueroa RE, Ginsberg LE, et al. Allergic fungal sinusitis: CT findings. Radiology 1998;207:417–22.

20. Plonk DP, Luong A. Current understanding of allergic fungal rhinosinusitis and treatment implications. Curr Opin Otolaryngol Head Neck Surg 2014;22:221–6.
21. Lund VJ, Milroy CM. Fronto-ethmoidal mucocoeles: a histopathological analysis. J Laryngol Otol 1991;105:921–3.
22. Stiernberg CM, Bailey BJ, Calhoun KH, et al. Management of invasive frontoethmoidal sinus mucoceles. Arch Otolaryngol Head Neck Surg 1986;112:1060–3.
23. Nomura K, Hidaka H, Arakawa K, et al. Outcomes of frontal mucoceles treated with conventional endoscopic sinus surgery. Acta Otolaryngol 2015;135:819–23.
24. Akiyama K, Karaki M, Mori N. Evaluation of adult Pott's puffy tumor: our five cases and 27 literature cases. Laryngoscope 2012;122:2382–8.
25. Walgama E, Ahn C, Batra PS. Surgical management of frontal sinus inverted papilloma: a systematic review. Laryngoscope 2012;122:1205–9.
26. Cooper JS, Porter K, Mallin K, et al. National Cancer Database report on cancer of the head and neck: 10-year update. Head Neck 2009;31:748–58.
27. Woodworth B, Schlosser R. Frontal Sinus Cerebrospinal Fluid Leaks. In: Kountakis S, Senior B, Draf W, editors. The frontal sinus. Heidelberg (Germany): Springer Berlin; 2005. p. 143–52.
28. Ramadan H. History of frontal sinus surgery. In: Kountakis S, Senior B, Draf W, editors. The frontal sinus. Heidelberg (Germany): Springer Berlin; 2005. p. 1–6.
29. Eloy JA, Friedel ME, Murray KP, et al. Modified hemi-Lothrop procedure for supraorbital frontal sinus access: a cadaveric feasibility study. Otolaryngol Head Neck Surg 2011;145:489–93.
30. Eloy JA, Kuperan AB, Friedel ME, et al. Modified hemi-Lothrop procedure for supraorbital frontal sinus access: a case series. Otolaryngol Head Neck Surg 2012;147:167–9.
31. Friedel ME, Li S, Langer PD, et al. Modified hemi-Lothrop procedure for supraorbital ethmoid lesion access. Laryngoscope 2012;122:442–4.
32. Liu JK, Mendelson ZS, Dubal PM, et al. The modified hemi-Lothrop procedure: a variation of the endoscopic endonasal approach for resection of a supraorbital psammomatoid ossifying fibroma. J Clin Neurosci 2014;21:2233–8.
33. Eloy JA, Friedel ME, Kuperan AB, et al. Modified mini-Lothrop/extended Draf IIB procedure for contralateral frontal sinus disease: a cadaveric feasibility study. Otolaryngol Head Neck Surg 2012;146:165–8.
34. Eloy JA, Friedel ME, Kuperan AB, et al. Modified mini-Lothrop/extended Draf IIB procedure for contralateral frontal sinus disease: a case series. Int Forum Allergy Rhinol 2012;2:321–4.
35. Eloy JA, Liu JK, Choudhry OJ, et al. Modified subtotal lothrop procedure for extended frontal sinus and anterior skull base access: a cadaveric feasibility study with clinical correlates. Journal of neurological surgery Part B. Skull base 2013;74:130–5.
36. Eloy JA, Mady LJ, Kanumuri VV, et al. Modified subtotal-Lothrop procedure for extended frontal sinus and anterior skull-base access: a case series. Int Forum Allergy Rhinol 2014;4:517–21.

Evaluation and Decision Making in Frontal Sinus Surgery

 CrossMark

Alok T. Saini, MD, Satish Govindaraj, MD*

KEYWORDS

- Frontal sinus outflow tract • Mucociliary clearance • Acute viral rhinosinusitis
- Acute bacterial rhinosinusitis • Chronic rhinosinusitis • Surgical decision making

KEY POINTS

- Management of frontal sinusitis requires a thorough understanding of the anatomy of the frontal sinus and its outflow tract and the pathogenesis of acute and chronic sinusitis.
- Each case of frontal sinusitis is unique and so requires an individualized approach for management.
- Knowledge of the surgical techniques available and the specific circumstances in which they should be used is necessary for obtaining optimal outcomes in the treatment of frontal sinusitis.

INTRODUCTION

Management of frontal sinusitis can be challenging for even the most experienced otolaryngologists. The challenges that the treating physician face are deciding whether medical or surgical treatment is needed and if a surgical procedure is necessary, then determining which procedure will serve as the best option. Many times there is no clear-cut solution, and the answer rests with the physician's clinical judgment and experience.

A thorough understanding of both the pathogenesis of acute and chronic rhinosinusitis (CRS) and the anatomy of the frontal sinus is required in order to properly treat frontal sinusitis and its complications. To the young otolaryngologist, simply understanding the complex anatomy of the frontal sinus and its outflow tract can be difficult. After years of training, frontal sinus surgery remains technically challenging to even the most skilled rhinologists; however, perhaps the most difficult aspect of managing frontal sinusitis is understanding the treatment options available and knowing which approach provides the highest likelihood of success in specific circumstances. When contemplating treatment, one must distinguish between acute and chronic

No conflicts or disclosures for either author.
Otolaryngology-Head and Neck Surgery, Mount Sinai Medical Center, One Gustave L. Levy Place, New York, NY 10029, USA
* Corresponding author.
E-mail address: satish.govindaraj@mountsinai.org

Otolaryngol Clin N Am 49 (2016) 911–925
http://dx.doi.org/10.1016/j.otc.2016.03.015   **oto.theclinics.com**
0030-6665/16/$ – see front matter © 2016 Elsevier Inc. All rights reserved.

Abbreviations	
CRS	Chronic rhinosinusitis
CT	Computed tomography
EMLP	Endoscopic modified Lothrop procedure
FSOT	Frontal sinus outflow tract
LP	Lothrop procedure
MMLP	Modified mini-Lothrop procedure
MSLP	Modified subtotal-Lothrop procedure

sinusitis. Once that distinction is made, medical and surgical treatment protocols can be initiated. These protocols are determined by severity of disease, patient anatomy, and technical expertise of the operating surgeon. These factors all come into play with both the evaluation and the decision making in frontal sinus surgery.

RELEVANT ANATOMY/PATHOPHYSIOLOGY
Anatomy

In most adults, 2 frontal sinuses exist and are separated by an intersinus septum that can vary in location. Each sinus consists of a thick anterior plate that serves as a buffer in the setting of trauma and a thinner posterior plate. The posterior plate separates the frontal sinus from the anterior cranial fossa, and below the frontal sinus floor is the orbit. For this reason, infection in the frontal sinus has the potential to spread to both the orbit and the intracranial cavity.

The frontal sinus outflow tract (FSOT) is described as an hourglass. It consists mainly of 3 structures: the frontal sinus infundibulum, ostium, and recess. The frontal sinus infundibulum is a funnel-shaped area at the inferior aspect of the frontal sinus that leads to the frontal sinus ostium. The ostium opens into the frontal sinus recess. The frontal recess is bounded laterally by the lamina papyracea, medially by the middle turbinate, anteriorly by the agger nasi, and posteriorly by the ethmoid bulla. The superior attachment of the uncinate process determines whether the frontal sinus has a medial or lateral drainage pathway. Most commonly, the uncinate attaches to the lamina papyracea, leading to a medial drainage pathway (**Fig. 1**). In cases where the uncinate attaches to the skull base, the frontal sinus drains lateral to the uncinate.

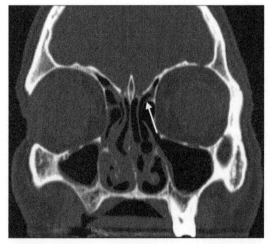

Fig. 1. Arrow demonstrates uncinate attaching to lamina papyracea signifying a medial frontal sinus drainage pathway.

Preoperative evaluation of the computed tomographic (CT) scan is in many ways the most critical aspect of surgical decision making for frontal sinus surgery. Identification of the drainage pathway helps direct a surgeon to dissect in a way that minimizes mucosal trauma. In addition, depending on frontal sinus aeration, a purely endoscopic approach may not be feasible or, if entertained, an extended approach such as a modified Lothrop procedure (LP) may be needed.

Many cells have been described that can obstruct the FSOT. Bent and colleagues[1] have described 4 types of frontal infundibular cells that can obstruct the anterior aspect of the FSOT. A type I frontal cell is an individual anterior ethmoid cell located superior to the agger nasi. Type II frontal cells consist of a tier of anterior ethmoid cells located superior to the agger nasi. A type III frontal cell is a cell arising superior to the agger nasi and extending into the frontal sinus. A type IV cell is an isolated cell arising within the frontal sinus. Other cells that can obstruct the posterior aspect of the FSOT include suprabullar and frontal bullar cells. The most common air cell in the frontal recess is the agger nasi that has variable degrees of posterior aeration. The more posterior it aerates, the further posterior the origin of the FSOT will be (**Fig. 2**).

Normal mucosal function, termed mucociliary clearance, plays a critical role in protecting the frontal sinus against infectious agents. The ciliated epithelium allows for coordinated movement of mucus through the sinus cavity, and mucociliary flow in the frontal sinus has been described to occur in a spiral pattern. Mucociliary flow progresses superiorly along the intersinus septum, laterally across the roof, and inferiorly along the lateral wall before traveling medially along the floor to drain into the frontal recess (**Fig. 3**). This concept is crucial to understand, and surgical techniques should be performed in a way that minimizes damage to the delicate ciliary apparatus and incorporates the mucociliary clearance pathway into the surgical approach.[2]

Pathophysiology

Rhinosinusitis is an inflammation of the nose and paranasal sinuses. It can be classified as acute or chronic. Acute sinusitis is defined as sinusitis lasting less than 4 weeks, whereas chronic sinusitis is defined as lasting greater than 12 weeks.

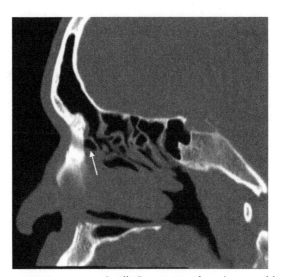

Fig. 2. Arrow demonstrates agger nasi cell. One can see how increased levels of posterior aeration could displace frontal recess outflow posteriorly.

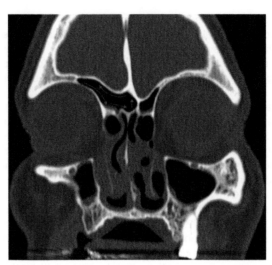

Fig. 3. Arrows demonstrate mucociliary flow through the frontal sinus. Mucus progresses in a coordinate fashion superiorly along the intersinus septum, laterally across the roof, and inferiorly along the lateral wall before traveling medially along the floor to drain into the frontal recess.

An exhaustive overview of the underlying pathogenesis of acute and CRS is outside the scope of this article. However, a brief review of the basic underlying mechanisms is discussed.

In acute frontal sinusitis, infectious causes predominate. Typically, a viral upper respiratory infection triggers an immunologic response. The ensuing inflammatory response results in mucosal edema in the nose and paranasal sinuses. Mucosal edema leads to ostium obstruction resulting in mucociliary stasis and bacterial overgrowth. In the frontal sinus, this may lead to the development of intracranial spread via retrograde thrombophlebitis through the diploic veins in the frontal bone known as the veins of Breschet[3]; this may lead to meningitis, brain abscess, or in severe cases, osteomyelitis of the frontal bone. Epidural extension of infection separates the dura mater from the inner table of the frontal bone; this interferes with the blood supply to this area and facilitates further spread of infection. Once the infection spreads beyond the dura to the brain, large brain abscesses may develop because glial tissue serves as a weak barrier to infection.[3] Epidural empyemas are often associated with acute osteomyelitis of the frontal bone, so when seen clinically, an assumption of osteomyelitis should be made. This entity, when associated with toxic appearance and tender swelling over the frontal bone, is called Pott's puffy tumor. Chronic osteomyelitis of the frontal bone presents as a lump on the head in the absence of a toxic appearance.

Most brain abscesses occur in the first 2 decades of life and are most often associated with frontal sinusitis. This age group is more susceptible to sinus infections. Surgical drainage of the intracranial process and paranasal sinuses is indicated in these cases.

In chronic sinusitis, several factors may predispose to mucosal inflammation, and there is no single, universally accepted mechanism underlying the disease process.

Defects at the mucosal level may allow for an aggressive immune response against the micro-organisms residing within the sinonasal cavity. The ensuing immune response can lead to mucosal inflammation, ostial obstruction, and bacterial overgrowth. Other contributing factors may include anatomic sources of obstruction (eg, septal deviation, concha bullosa, frontal cells), immune deficiencies, ciliary motility disorders, or allergies.

CLINICAL PRESENTATION/EXAMINATION/DIAGNOSIS

Acute viral sinusitis is diagnosed in patients with purulent nasal discharge along with nasal obstruction and/or facial pain-pressure-fullness lasting less than 4 weeks. Acute bacterial sinusitis is diagnosed when symptoms last greater than 10 days or when symptoms acutely worsen within 10 days after an initial period of improvement (**Table 1**).[4]

Acute frontal sinusitis is most common in adolescent men, and it is commonly preceded by an upper respiratory illness. The most common symptom in acute frontal sinusitis is frontal headache. One should consider the diagnosis in anyone with signs of acute rhinosinusitis and frontal headache. In addition, the diagnosis should be considered in anyone with no prior history of headaches who develops new onset frontal headache.[5] No diagnostic criteria specific for frontal sinusitis exists; rather, the criteria for diagnosing acute sinusitis are used, and involvement of the frontal sinus is assessed based on symptomatology and examination findings.

On nasal endoscopy, purulent drainage in the frontal recess indicates involvement of the frontal sinus but is not always present. When possible, cultures should be obtained to guide antimicrobial therapy. In uncomplicated cases of acute sinusitis, imaging is not required to confirm the diagnosis.

Orbital complications are more likely to arise from the ethmoid cells but can develop from the frontal sinus due to its proximity to the orbital roof. Intracranial complications such as epidural abscess, subdural abscess, and meningitis can present with subtle findings; therefore, a high index of suspicion is necessary for early and accurate diagnosis of these complications. Patients may complain of lethargy, change in personality, or in severe cases, seizures with severe headache or generally toxic appearance. Other signs may include periorbital edema or erythema, extraocular movement restrictions, vision changes, nausea, vomiting, altered mental status, photophobia, or neurologic deficits.

Diagnosis of acute frontal sinusitis can be confirmed with CT scan of the sinuses. In cases where extrasinus spread to the orbit or brain is suspected, an MRI with and without contrast is indicated.

Table 1 Diagnostic criteria for acute sinusitis		
Acute rhinosinusitis	<4 wk of purulent nasal drainage with nasal obstruction and/or facial pain/pressure	—
Acute viral rhinosinusitis	Symptoms present <10 d	Symptoms not worsening
Acute bacterial rhinosinusitis	Symptoms present >10 d	Symptoms worsening after initial improvement

Adapted from Rosenfeld RM, Piccirillo JF, Chandrasekhar SS, et al. Clinical practice guideline (update): adult sinusitis. Otolaryngol Head Neck Surg 2015;152(2 Suppl):S1–39.

Treatment of complicated acute frontal sinusitis includes aggressive medical and surgical management. Appropriate cultures should be obtained if possible. In the event of meningitis, an LP may be obtained after CT confirms the lack of an intracranial mass or space-occupying process. Following these diagnostic measures, broad spectrum intravenous antibiotics should be initiated. Surgical treatment of the frontal sinus is necessary either via frontal sinus trephination, via endoscopic frontal sinusotomy, or both. Endoscopic frontal sinusotomy is more difficult to perform in the acutely inflamed sinus and is often delayed in this setting.

CRS is diagnosed in patients with 2 or more of the following: nasal obstruction, purulent nasal drainage (rhinorrhea or postnasal drip), anosmia/hyposmia, and facial fullness-pressure-pain lasting longer than 12 weeks in addition to either radiographic evidence of sinusitis, purulent nasal drainage, or middle meatus edema or polyps. CRS can further be classified as chronic sinusitis with polyposis and chronic sinusitis without polyposis; the mechanisms underlying the development of each seem to be distinct.[4]

Most patients with chronic frontal sinusitis do not have isolated frontal disease. However, chronic frontal sinusitis is diagnosed in patients with CRS who are found to have involvement of the frontal sinus. In addition, certain pathologies may predispose patients to developing isolated frontal disease. Examples include the presence of frontal sinus osteomas, mucoceles, or tumors that obstruct the FSOT. In addition, many patients who have previously undergone functional endoscopic sinus surgery may continue to have or may develop chronic frontal sinusitis as a result of neo-osteogenesis or scarring resulting in a narrowed FSOT. Aberrations in technique and/or complications of healing are often responsible for iatrogenic cases.

Diagnosis can be confirmed with nasal endoscopy. The use of angled endoscopes (30°, 45°, and 70°) allows for the evaluation of the frontal sinus and its outflow tract in most patients. It is important to note the presence or absence of the middle turbinate and its location, scarring or synechiae from previous operations, and the location of any polyps. In addition, CT of the paranasal sinuses using thin (<3 mm) cuts is a necessary adjunct. It is common practice to obtain imaging only after the patient has completed a course of aggressive medical management unless complications are suspected. MRI may be particularly useful to evaluate suspected orbital or intracranial extension. Thorough review of all imaging with careful attention paid to the FSOT is absolutely crucial to identify factors leading to the development of frontal sinusitis. Particular attention should be paid to the size and pneumatization of the frontal sinus, the presence of any anatomic abnormalities predisposing to frontal sinusitis (eg, frontal cells, supraorbital cells, suprabullar cells, intersinus septal cells, osteomas, or other benign tumors involving the frontal sinus), the anterior-posterior dimension from the nasal root to the anterior cranial fossa including the nasal beak, the presence or absence of the middle turbinate or its remnant, and the attachment site of the uncinate. The frontal recess anatomy dictates the choice of surgical approach necessary to treat the frontal sinus.

THERAPEUTIC PROCEDURES
Medical Management of Acute Frontal Sinusitis

Treatment of uncomplicated acute frontal sinusitis is primarily medical and consists of antibiotics, nasal saline, and nasal decongestants. In certain patients, steroids may be useful in reducing mucosal edema and ostial obstruction, especially in the polyp patient suffering from an acute exacerbation of frontal sinusitis. Surgical therapy is rarely necessary in uncomplicated cases (**Fig. 4**).

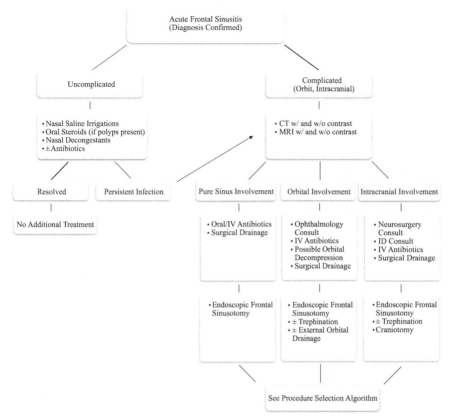

Fig. 4. Algorithm for management of acute frontal sinusitis. ID, infectious disease; IV, intravenous.

Medical Management of Chronic Frontal Sinusitis

Generally, aggressive medical management is considered to be first-line treatment for CRS, including cases with frontal sinus involvement. A combination of oral antibiotics, oral steroids, nasal saline sprays or irrigations, and topical steroid sprays or irrigations is considered to be the mainstay of therapy. However, many patients will continue to remain symptomatic despite maximal medical therapy. Patients who remain symptomatic may benefit from surgical intervention. The type of surgical intervention necessary is determined on an individual basis.

Surgical Management of Frontal Sinusitis

When medical therapy fails, surgical treatment of inflammatory frontal sinus disease is indicated. Surgical decision making with respect to the ideal approach to the frontal sinus can be a challenge. Hence, a thorough understanding of the available surgical techniques and the specific circumstances in which each is most effective is critical. The surgical approaches mentioned in the following section are described in detail elsewhere in the text. The focus here remains on understanding the set of circumstances in which each procedure should be used **(Fig. 5)**.

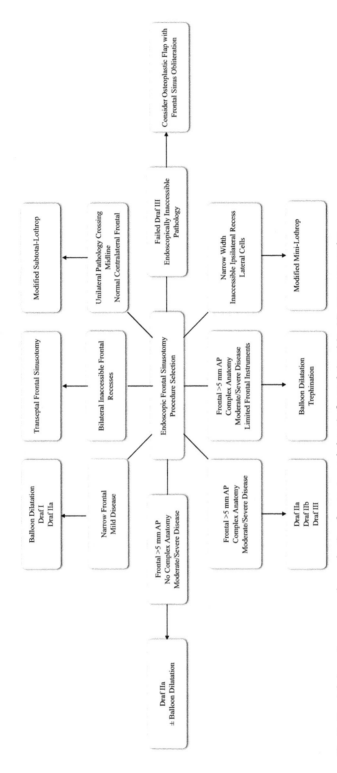

Fig. 5. Frontal sinusotomy procedure selection for acute and chronic frontal sinusitis. AP, anteroposterior.

Draf Types I–III

Draf[6] classified 3 types of endoscopic frontal sinus drainage. Type I involves an anterior ethmoidectomy, including the frontal recess but sparing the frontal sinus infundibulum and ostia. Type IIa additionally involves resection of the floor of the frontal sinus from the lamina papyracea laterally to the middle turbinate medially. Type IIb differs only in that the medial boundary of dissection is the nasal septum rather than the middle turbinate. Type III involves resection of the anterior superior aspect of the nasal septum as well as the inferior portion of the frontal intersinus septum in addition to bilateral type IIb procedures.

Generally, Draf type I should be considered in patients with minimal, asymptomatic frontal sinus inflammation. Frontal sinus balloon dilatation is an option in this setting as well, especially in the case where the surgeon does not feel comfortable dissecting in the frontal recess or when the anatomy of the frontal sinus is very narrow and any scarring may result in outflow obstruction. With improved instrumentation and surgical techniques, most cases of frontal sinusitis are managed with a Draf IIa frontal sinusotomy, which is discussed later.

Draf type IIa is indicated for primary and revision cases in which persistent chronic frontal sinusitis is attributable to remnant uncinate, agger nasi, or frontal recess cells and is the workhorse endoscopic procedure for the frontal sinus. It can also be used to treat medially located benign tumors and mucoceles. In addition, it can be used in cases of complicated acute frontal sinusitis along with trephination.

The indications for Draf type IIb are the same as those for Draf type IIa. Type IIb should be considered in cases where an osteitic middle turbinate or a frontal intersinus septal cell is thought to be contributing to the disease process. Resecting the floor medially will allow incorporation of that cell into the frontal sinus. In addition, Draf type IIb should be performed if the resulting ostium after Draf type IIa is less than 5 mm in diameter.[7,8]

Draf type III, also known as the endoscopic modified Lothrop procedure (EMLP), is indicated for cases that have failed multiple attempts at surgical therapy, including failed obliterations via osteoplastic flap approach.[9–11] It should be strongly considered in primary cases with poor prognostic factors, such as polyposis, aspirin sensitivity, asthma, ciliary motility disorders, and immunocompromised states.[8] It can be used for mucoceles[12] or complicated frontal sinusitis with intracranial or orbital involvement.[10] It is also indicated in cases of benign and malignant tumors and is particularly useful in these cases because it ensures easy access for endoscopic tumor surveillance postoperatively. Generally, one should give consideration to type III drainage any time the use of an osteoplastic flap is contemplated. Success rates for achieving patent frontal sinus ostia have reportedly been as high as 93%.[13] The authors' preferred approach has been the outside-in approach described by Chin and colleagues.[14]

Notably, Draf type III should be avoided if the frontal sinus or frontal recess is hypoplastic, if the anterior-posterior dimension between the nasal bones at the nasal root and the anterior skull base (including the frontal beak) is less than 1.5 cm, or if the nasal beak is greater than 1 cm in anterior-posterior thickness.[13,15,16]

Transseptal Frontal Sinusotomy

Transseptal frontal sinusotomy has similar indications to Draf type III but is particularly useful in cases of chronic frontal sinusitis when the frontal recess cannot be cannulated (often due to neo-osteogenesis or a lateralized middle turbinate remnant). The procedure is based on the stable relationship between the nasal septum and the midline floor of the frontal sinus, which provides a safe entry point into the frontal sinus. A relative contraindication is an anterior-to-posterior diameter of less than 1.2 cm.[17,18]

Modified Mini-Lothrop/Extended Draf IIb

More recently, a modification to the standard Draf type IIb, the extended Draf type IIb or modified mini-Lothrop (MMLP), has been described. It affords access to the ipsilateral frontal sinus via a contralateral approach and can be used in frontal sinus disease that cannot be approached using traditional endoscopic technique on the ipsilateral side. This approach can be particularly useful in situations with irreversible obstruction of the frontal sinus, such as iatrogenic or traumatic scarring, frontal recess stenosis, tumor, or prior medial orbital wall decompression. Use of this technique may be an alternative to a combined trephination/endoscopic approach and may avoid more extensive procedures such as a Draf type III, transseptal frontal sinusotomy, or osteoplastic flap.[19]

Modified Subtotal-Lothrop

A similar modification to the standard Draf type IIb, the modified subtotal-Lothrop (MSLP), has been described. This procedure serves as a surgical option in the setting of unilateral chronic frontal sinusitis (also an option for unilateral tumors such as inverted papilloma or osteoma) with cells or a sinus that crosses the midline and a normal contralateral frontal recess. In contrast to the MMLP, this procedure approaches the diseased frontal sinus via an ipsilateral approach. Rather than performing a traditional EMLP, one preserves the contralateral (disease-free) frontal sinus and recess. This technique allows preservation of the normally functioning frontal sinus while providing adequate surgical access to the diseased frontal sinus.[20]

Frontal Trephination

Frontal trephination, or mini-trephination, is most commonly used for cases of complicated acute frontal sinusitis because it creates a drainage pathway for the acutely infected frontal sinus and serves as a means of catheter placement for irrigation **(Fig. 6)**. Although an endoscopic frontal sinusotomy may adequately drain the frontal sinus, in the acutely infected condition, it is more difficult to perform. Often the frontal recess is acutely inflamed, edematous, and obstructed solely from mucosal edema. The decision to perform an endoscopic frontal sinusotomy in this setting depends on the surgical expertise of the operating physician. Treatment of associated

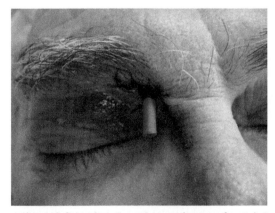

Fig. 6. Red rubber catheter left in place in patient with acute frontal sinusitis complicated by epidural abscess. Sinus irrigation can be performed through catheter to maintain patency of frontal sinus outflow tract.

complications may require simultaneous orbital decompression, drainage of an intra-orbital abscess, or craniotomy for drainage of an intracranial abscess.

Frontal trephination can also be used as an adjunct to endoscopic frontal sinusotomy in cases where pathology is inaccessible via endoscopic techniques or where the frontal sinus cannot be cannulated using endoscopic techniques.[21,22] This combined approach may allow laterally based mucoceles or frontal cells to be drained without the need for an extensive external approach. It can also be useful in cases with severely distorted anatomy precluding safe identification or entry into the frontal sinus using endoscopic techniques alone. Other indications for the combined approach are large tumors such as osteomas, fibrous dysplasia, and inverted papillomas.[23]

Frontal Sinus Rescue Procedure

The frontal sinus rescue procedure, also known as the frontal sinusotomy with muco-periosteal flap advancement, can be used in cases of persistent or recurrent chronic frontal sinusitis due to a lateralized or collapsed middle turbinate remnant. It involves resection of the bony and soft tissue obstruction caused by the middle turbinate and uses a small mucoperiosteal flap to cover the resulting exposed bone to prevent neo-osteogenesis. The procedure is advantageous because it preserves the lateral mucosa of the frontal sinus recess (which is responsible for mucus clearance) and is less invasive than alternatives such as the Draf type III or osteoplastic flap.[24,25]

External Frontoethmoidectomy

No discussion of the surgical management of the frontal sinus would be complete without the mention of the Lynch procedure, or external frontoethmoidectomy, because it was once considered the workhorse operation for chronic frontal sinusitis. However, in regard to frontal sinusitis alone, the procedure has largely been replaced by the aforementioned less invasive, endoscopic techniques. Although the external frontoethmoidectomy has limited indications, an example of its utility is the case of acute frontal sinusitis complicated with an orbital abscess. This approach allows drainage of the frontal sinus as well as the abscess in the setting of a surgical field that does not allow a safe endoscopic frontal sinusotomy to be performed. In addition, it can be used in the treatment of orbital complications from endoscopic surgery or in cases of extensive frontal sinus tumors. The disadvantage is that the FSOT needs to be managed with a stent or close postoperative monitoring because the orbital contents can herniate medially and obstruct the frontal outflow.

Osteoplastic Flap

The osteoplastic flap with or without frontal sinus obliteration is indicated in cases of chronic frontal sinusitis failing previous endoscopic and/or open procedures where Draf type III cannot be performed or in cases of Draf type III failure. In addition, it can be used in the setting of chronic frontal sinusitis with marked neo-osteogenesis or acute frontal sinusitis with associated osteomyelitis of the frontal bone that requires bone debridement. It is particularly useful for laterally based pathology (mucoceles, frontal cells, or osteomas) that is otherwise inaccessible via endoscopic techniques.[26–31]

Table 2 summarizes the clinical indications and contraindications for the various surgical approaches.

OUTCOMES

The outcomes for both primary and revision endoscopic frontal sinus surgery have been encouraging. Naidoo and colleagues[32] reported the outcomes of primary frontal

Table 2
Summary of clinical indications and contraindications for various approaches to the frontal sinus

Procedure	Indication	Contraindication
Frontal sinus balloon dilatation	Mild to moderate chronic frontal sinusitis	Dehiscence of the skull base, posterior table of frontal sinus, or orbit
Draf type I	Primary treatment of asymptomatic, mild chronic frontal sinusitis refractory to medical management	—
Draf type IIa	1. Primary acute or chronic frontal sinusitis 2. Failed Draf type I or balloon sinusotomy 3. Medially located benign tumors and mucoceles	—
Draf type IIb	1. All indications of Draf IIa 2. CRS with osteitic middle turbinate or frontal intersinus septal cell 3. Draf IIa with resulting ostia <5 mm	—
Draf type III/EMLP	1. Failed multiple surgical interventions (either endoscopic or open) 2. Primary CRS cases with polyposis, asthma, aspirin sensitivity, immunocompromised states, ciliary motility disorders 3. Unobliterated frontal sinus with medially located mucocele 4. Benign and select malignant tumors	1. Anterior-posterior dimension of nasal root to anterior cranial fossa <5 mm 2. Nasal beak >1 cm[a] 3. Hypoplastic frontal sinus or frontal recess
Transeptal frontal sinusotomy	All indications for Draf III but particularly useful for cases in which the frontal recess cannot be cannulated endonasally	Anterior-posterior dimension of nasal root to anterior cranial fossa <1.2 cm[a]
MMLP	Unilateral frontal CRS with inaccessible ipsilateral frontal sinus but accessible contralateral frontal sinus	—
MSLP	Unilateral frontal CRS with cells that cross midline and a normal contralateral frontal sinus	—
Frontal trephination	Complicated acute frontal sinusitis	—
Frontal trephination with endonasal approach	1. Laterally based mucoceles or frontal cells 2. Inability to easily identify frontal recess endonasally 3. Complicated acute frontal sinusitis (Draf I–III)	—
Osteoplastic flap	1. Failed multiple surgical interventions (either endoscopic or open) 2. Laterally based pathology (mucoceles, osteomas, tumors)	—

[a] These dimensions are relative contraindications. Whether to proceed with one of these approaches is based on expertise and experience of surgeon if done with dimensions that are less than described.

sinus surgery for 109 patients who underwent Draf IIa. They found that the overall patency rate was 92%, and complete symptom resolution occurred in 78% of patients with average follow-up of 16.2 months. In addition, reported long-term outcomes for revision cases have also been promising. Batra and colleagues[33] reported the results of 30 frontal sinus drill-out procedures (including Draf IIb, Draf III, and transeptal frontal sinusotomy). Twenty-six cases were revision cases. They found that endoscopic patency of the neo-ostium occurred in 92% of cases and that symptoms resolved or improved in 88% of cases with average follow-up of 16.3 months. Naidoo and colleagues[34] reported on 229 patients who had undergone an average of 3.8 previous procedures who underwent revision surgery with the EMLP/Draf III. They found that the procedure was successful in 95% of cases because no further surgical intervention was required. They noted that allergic fungal sinusitis and recurrent *Staphylococcal aureus* infections were potential risk factors for surgical failure. Other risk factors for failure include advanced degrees of preoperative disease (partial or total opacification of the sinus as opposed to mucosal thickening alone) and prior failed surgical intervention.[35] A systematic review and meta-analysis reported outcomes on the EMLP. They reviewed 18 studies that included 612 patients. They found the rate of major and minor complications to be less than 1% and 4%, respectively. They ultimately included 394 patients for outcome analysis. They demonstrated partial or complete frontal sinus patency in 95.9% of cases and noted improvement of symptoms in 82.2% of patients with average follow-up of 28.5 months. The overall failure rate, defined as need for further surgery, was 13.9%. Notably, among the failures, 80% underwent revision EMLP and only 20% required osteoplastic frontal sinus obliteration.[36] Overall, results are demonstrating that the range of endoscopic frontal sinus surgery appears to be safe and efficacious.

SUMMARY

Management of frontal sinusitis requires a thorough understanding of the anatomy of the frontal sinus and its outflow tract and the pathogenesis of acute and chronic sinusitis. Each case of frontal sinusitis is unique and so requires an individualized approach for management. Knowledge of the surgical techniques available and the specific circumstances in which they should be used is necessary for obtaining optimal outcomes in the treatment of frontal sinusitis.

REFERENCES

1. Bent JP, Cuilty-Siller C, Kuhn FA. The frontal cell as a cause of frontal sinus obstruction. Am J Rhinol 1994;8:185–91.
2. Messerklinger W. On the drainage of the normal frontal sinus of man. Acta Otolaryngol 1967;63(2):176–81.
3. Osei-Yeboah C, Neequaye J, Bulley H, et al. Osteomyelitis of the frontal bone. Ghana Med J 2007;41(2):88–90.
4. Rosenfeld RM, Piccirillo JF, Chandrasekhar SS, et al. Clinical practice guideline (update): adult sinusitis. Otolaryngol Head Neck Surg 2015;152(2 Suppl):S1–39.
5. Winther B, Gwaltney J. Microbiology of chronic frontal sinusitis. In: Kountakis SE, Senior BA, Draf W, editors. The frontal sinus. Heidelberg (Germany): Springer; 2005. p. 53–6.
6. Draf W. Endonasal micro-endoscopic frontal sinus surgery: the Fulda concept. Op Tech Otolaryngol Head Neck Surg 1991;2:234–40.

7. Chou AG, Kennedy DW. Revision endoscopic frontal sinus surgery. In: Kountakis SE, Senior BA, Draf W, editors. The frontal sinus. Heidelberg (Germany): Springer; 2005. p. 191–9.
8. Draf W. Endonasal frontal sinus drainage type I-III according to Draf. In: Kountakis SE, Senior BA, Draf W, editors. The frontal sinus. Heidelberg (Germany): Springer; 2005. p. 220–31.
9. Becker DG, Moore D, Lindsey WH, et al. Modified transnasal endoscopic Lothrop procedure: further considerations. Laryngoscope 1995;105(11):1161–6.
10. Wormald PJ, Ananda A, Nair S. Modified endoscopic Lothrop as a salvage for the failed osteoplastic flap with obliteration. Laryngoscope 2003;113(11):1988–92.
11. Gross WE, Gross CW, Becker D, et al. Modified transnasal endoscopic Lothrop procedure as an alternative to frontal sinus obliteration. Otolaryngol Head Neck Surg 1995;113(4):427–34.
12. Khong JJ, Malhotra R, Selva D, et al. Efficacy of endoscopic sinus surgery for paranasal sinus mucocele including modified endoscopic Lothrop procedure for frontal sinus mucocele. J Laryngal Otol 2004;118(5):352–6.
13. Wormald PJ. Salvage frontal sinus surgery: the endoscopic modified Lothrop procedure. Laryngoscope 2003;113(2):276–83.
14. Chin D, Snidvongs K, Kaslish L, et al. The outside-in approach to the modified endoscopic Lothrop procedure. Laryngoscope 2012;122(8):1661–9.
15. Kountakis SE. Endoscopic modified Lothrop procedure. In: Kountakis SE, Senior BA, Draf W, editors. The frontal sinus. Heidelberg (Germany): Springer; 2005. p. 233–41.
16. Gross CW, Schlosser RJ. The modified Lothrop procedure: lessons learned. Laryngoscope 2001;111(7):1302–5.
17. Batra PS, Lanza DC. Endoscopic trans-septal frontal sinusotomy. In: Kountakis SE, Senior BA, Draf W, editors. The frontal sinus. Heidelberg (Germany): Springer; 2005. p. 251–9.
18. McLaughlin RB, Hwang PH, Lanza DC. Endoscopic trans-septal frontal sinusotomy: the rationale and results of an alternative technique. Am J Rhinol 1999;13(4):279–87.
19. Eloy JA, Frieden ME, Kuperan AB, et al. Modified mini-Lothrop/extended Draf IIB procedure for contralateral frontal sinus disease: a case series. Int Forum Allergy Rhinol 2012;2(4):321–4.
20. Eloy JA, Mady LJ, Kanumuri VV, et al. Modified subtotal-Lothrop procedure for extended frontal sinus and anterior skull base access: a case series. Int Forum Allergy Rhinol 2014;4(6):517–21.
21. Patel AM, Vaughan WC. "Above and below" FESS: simple trephine with endoscopic sinus surgery. In: Kountakis SE, Senior BA, Draf W, editors. The frontal sinus. Heidelberg (Germany): Springer; 2005. p. 211–8.
22. Bent JP, Spears RA, Kuhn FA, et al. Combined endoscopic intranasal and external frontal sinusotomy. Am J Rhinol 1997;11(5):349–54.
23. Gallagher RM, Gross CW. The role of mini-trephination in the management of frontal sinusitis. Am J Rhinol 1999;13(4):289–93.
24. Kuhn FA, Javer AR, Nagpal K, et al. The frontal sinus rescue procedure: early experience and three-year follow up. Am J Rhinol 2000;14(4):211–6.
25. Citardi MJ, Javer AR, Kuhn FA. Revision endoscopic frontal sinusotomy with mucoperiosteal flap advancement: the frontal sinus rescue procedure. Otolaryng Clin North Am 2001;34(1):123–32.
26. Bockmuhl U. Osteoplastic frontal sinusotomy and reconstruction of frontal defects. In: Kountakis SE, Senior BA, Draf W, editors. The frontal sinus. Heidelberg (Germany): Springer; 2005. p. 281–8.

27. Weber R, Draf W, Keerl R, et al. Osteoplastic frontal sinus surgery with fat obliteration: technique and long-term results using magnetic resonance imaging in 82 operations. Laryngoscope 2000;110(6):1037–44.

28. Draf W, Weber R, Keerl R, et al. Current aspects of frontal sinus surgery. I: endonasal frontal sinus drainage in inflammatory disease of the paranasal sinuses. HNO 1995;43(6):352–7.

29. Weber R, Draf W, Keerl R, et al. Current aspects of frontal sinus surgery. II: external frontal sinus operation—osteoplastic approach. HNO 1995;43(6):358–63.

30. Weber R, Draf W, Keerl R, et al. Aspects of frontal sinus surgery. III: indications and results of osteoplastic frontal sinus operation. HNO 1995;43(7):414–20.

31. Hardy JM, Montgomery WW. Osteoplastic frontal sinusotomy: an analysis of 250 operations. Ann Otol Rhinol Laryngal 1976;85(4 Pt 1):523–32.

32. Naidoo Y, Wen D, Bassiouni A, et al. Long-term results after primary frontal sinus surgery. Int Forum Allergy Rhinol 2012;2(3):185–90.

33. Batra PS, Cannady SB, Lanza DC. Surgical outcomes of drill out procedures for complex frontal sinus pathology. Laryngoscope 2007;117(5):927–31.

34. Naidoo Y, Bassiouni A, Keen M, et al. Long-term outcomes for the endoscopic modified Lothrop/Draf III procedure: a 10-year review. Laryngoscope 2014; 124(1):43–9.

35. Chandra RK, Palmer JN, Tangsujarittham T, et al. Factors associated with failure of frontal sinusotomy in the early follow-up period. Otolaryngol Head Neck Surg 2004;131(4):514–8.

36. Anderson P, Sindwani R. Safety and efficacy of the endoscopic modified Lothrop procedure: a systematic review and meta-analysis. Laryngoscope 2009;119(9): 1828–33.

Medical Management of Frontal Sinusitis

Maheep Sohal, MD[a], Belachew Tessema, MD[a,b], Seth M. Brown, MD, MBA[a,b],*

KEYWORDS

- Frontal sinus • Medical management • Rhinosinusitis • Sinusitis • Pharmacotherapy

KEY POINTS

- Frontal sinusitis is a diverse entity that requires identification of the unique disease process to implement appropriate treatment.
- Isolated acute bacterial frontal sinusitis occurs primarily in adolescents and young adults secondary to pneumatization of the frontal sinuses and requires aggressive medical therapy and sometimes surgery to avoid complications.
- Intranasal corticosteroids have proved an effective long-term treatment of both acute and chronic frontal sinusitis.
- Oral corticosteroids are a powerful adjuvant in the treatment of chronic frontal sinusitis, especially for chronic frontal sinusitis with nasal polyposis.
- The use of bioabsorbable steroid-eluting stents, although currently not Food and Drug Administration approved for the frontal sinus, holds considerable promise for the maintenance of frontal sinus ostial patency.

INTRODUCTION

Rhinosinusitis is a term that has long been used to describe a diverse disease entity that encompasses several related but distinct conditions involving the paranasal sinuses. These distinctions are based on several factors, including chronicity, presence of polyposis, pathogens involved, and, of particular pertinence to this discussion, the specific sinus involved. Frontal sinusitis represents one such disease process with its own unique treatment considerations. Like rhinosinusitis as a whole, the role of medical management in the treatment of frontal sinusitis cannot be overlooked. To better understand both the indications and limitations of medical management, however, it is of paramount importance to recognize the various presentations of frontal sinus disease and the unique treatment consideration of those specific manifestations.

---

[a] Division of Otolaryngology, Department of Surgery, University of Connecticut School of Medicine, Farmington, CT, USA; [b] The Connecticut Sinus Institute, 21 South Road, Suite 112, Farmington, CT 06032, USA
* Corresponding author.
E-mail address: sethmbrown@msn.com

Otolaryngol Clin N Am 49 (2016) 927–934
http://dx.doi.org/10.1016/j.otc.2016.03.016
0030-6665/16/$ – see front matter © 2016 Elsevier Inc. All rights reserved.

oto.theclinics.com

ACUTE FRONTAL SINUSITIS

Sinusitis, as defined by the American Academy of Otolaryngology–Head and Neck Surgery Task Force on Rhinosinusitis, is an inflammatory disease of the paranasal sinuses with several major and minor criteria required for diagnosis.[1] Acute rhinosinusitis, more specifically, is defined by up to 4 weeks of sinonasal symptomatology.[2] The chronicity of disease, or lack thereof, has ramifications in regard to the likely pathogens involved. Acute frontal sinusitis typically occurs in the context of a recent or concurrent upper respiratory infection. As such, the most likely pathogens are viral and treatment is largely supportive, aimed at improving sinonasal drainage.

Microbiology

Acute bacterial frontal sinusitis, on the other hand, typically occurs in the context of a more diffuse process with involvement of other paranasal sinuses and is suggested by failure to respond to conservative management in a timely fashion. Isolated acute bacterial frontal sinusitis is an uncommon entity when viewed in the larger context of sinonasal disease and most commonly occurs in the adolescent or young adult population. This is thought to be due to the rapid pneumatization of the frontal sinuses that occurs between 6 and 20 years of age and is elaborated on later.[3] Studies evaluating the bacteriology of acute bacterial frontal sinus infections have typically shown *Haemophilus influenzae*, *Streptococcus pneumoniae*, and *Moraxella catarrhalis* as the causative organisms.[4] In this regard, antimicrobial management of acute frontal sinusitis does not dramatically differ from that of acute maxillary sinusitis.[5] The increasing incidence of penicillin resistant and β-lactamase–producing bacterial colonies has subsequent ramifications on antimicrobial therapy.

Antibiotic Therapy

For those patients who meet indications for antimicrobial therapy, treatment of acute bacterial frontal sinusitis must be targeted towards these commonly cultured microbes. Several evidence-based antibiotic treatment guidelines have been published and recommended amoxicillin with or without clavulanate for 5 to 10 days as a viable first-line option.[6,7] The decision to opt for amoxicillin-clavulanate versus amoxicillin alone is based on several factors, such as patient age, preceding antibiotic use, severity of infection, and underlying health. To optimize therapy, local resistance patterns must also be taken into account and may influence the decision to expand coverage. Other options for antibiotic therapy include either second-generation or third-generation cephalosporins as well as fluoroquinolones. Additionally, for penicillin-allergic patients, options include doxycycline and fluoroquinolones. Ideally, antimicrobial therapy should be culture directed and consideration should always be given to obtaining endoscopically guided sinonasal cultures.

Adjuvant Therapy

In addition to antibiotics, medical management for acute bacterial frontal sinusitis should be aimed at improving sinus ventilation and drainage. Adjuvant pharmacotherapy includes decongestants, mucolytics, nasal saline, and corticosteroids. Decongestants, whether systemic or intranasal, result in mucosal vasoconstriction and thus improve drainage via the frontal sinus drainage tract and the ostiomeatal complex. Intranasal decongestants, however, avoid the systemic side effects of α-agonists while offering superior nasal mucosal decongestion.[8] Care should be taken to avoid prolonged courses of topical decongestant given the risk of rhinitis medicamentosa. Nasal saline solutions have also been demonstrated to improve mucocilliary clearance, with hypertonic saline solutions specifically shown to increase nasal airway patency.[9,10] Expectorants, such as guaifenesin, are another adjuvant for improved mucus clearance and symptomatic treatment but, admittedly, with limited clinical evidence supporting their use.

Corticosteroids

In contrast, the role of corticosteroids in acute rhinosinusitis has been studied thoroughly. Ultimately, the utility of corticosteroids in the context of acute frontal sinusitis depends on the mechanism of delivery. Several meta-analyses have been performed to evaluate the impact of both intranasal and systemic delivery of corticosteroid both as monotherapy and in combination with antibiotic therapy. Whereas intranasal corticosteroid therapy has demonstrated success in reducing symptomatology in acute sinusitis, with a relatively benign side-effect profile, systemic corticosteroid therapy has not.[11] Systemic corticosteroids were not shown effective as monotherapy and demonstrated only modest symptom relief when used in conjunction with antibiotic therapy.[12] Additionally, the use of systemic corticosteroids inherently bears an increased risk of side effects not shared by intranasal delivery. In the context of acute frontal sinusitis, intranasal corticosteroids can be used as a useful adjuvant pharmacotherapy with systemic corticosteroids playing a limited role.

Pediatric Population

As discussed previously, frontal sinusitis has an increased incidence in the pediatric population, coinciding with the development of the frontal sinuses. In light of this, medical management of acute bacterial frontal sinusitis in pediatric patients warrants special attention. Given the location of the frontal sinuses, as well as the their relationship with the valveless diploic veins, untreated frontal sinusitis can lead to significant morbidity and even mortality. Acute bacterial frontal sinusitis in pediatric or young adult patients requires aggressive treatment to avoid such complications. Although complicated cases often fall within the realm of surgical management, uncomplicated cases – those without intracranial extension or abscess formation – can often be treated medically in the form of antibiotics, topical corticosteroids, and decongestants. Depending on the severity of disease, intravenous antibiotics and short courses of systemic steroids also may be warranted. Vigilance against the progression of frontal sinusitis is of the utmost importance to avoid delaying any potentially needed surgical intervention.

CHRONIC FRONTAL SINUSITIS

Whereas acute rhinosinusitis is defined by the presence of 4 weeks or fewer of symptoms, chronic rhinosinusitis is defined by 12 or more weeks of symptoms.[1] Like acute frontal sinusitis, the chronicity of symptoms has implications regarding the microbiology of chronic frontal sinus infections and, as a result, the medical management.

Antibiotic Therapy

Studies evaluating the bacteriology in chronic frontal sinusitis have demonstrated the existence of a wide variety of microbes, including gram-negative rods, such as *Pseudomonas aeruginosa*, anaerobes, coagulase-positive staphylococci and coagulase-negative staphylococci, and streptococci.[13] On this basis, initial antibiotic therapy for chronic frontal sinusitis does not significantly differ from that for acute bacterial frontal sinusitis, with amoxicillin with clavulanate providing adequate coverage on an empiric basis, albeit for longer initial durations. Although the microbiology of acute bacterial frontal sinusitis lends itself to narrow-spectrum antimicrobial therapy, antibiotic therapy for either initial medical management or acute exacerbations of chronic frontal sinusitis may require broader-spectrum therapy and also may be more likely to result in treatment failures. In addition, current research has suggested an increasing prevalence of methicillin-resistant strains of *Staphylococcus*, thus further stressing the importance of culture-directed antibiotics, especially in an era of growing concern over antibiotic resistance.[14,15]

Multiple investigations into novel antibiotic regimens for use in chronic sinusitis have also been performed. Although long-term antibiotic therapy is not recommended for chronic frontal sinusitis, there is some debate regarding the utility of long-term macrolide antibiotic administration given their unique anti-inflammatory and immunomodulatory effects. Low-dose daily macrolide therapy has been shown to inhibit the predominantly neutrophilic inflammation seen in chronic sinusitis without polyposis in vitro. Ultimately, although this may lead to modest improvement in select patients, further study is necessary and current literature is limited.[16] Similarly, topical antibiotic administration has also been debated. Thus far, studies into topical delivery of antibiotics, via either solution or nebulization, have not demonstrated statistically significant clinical improvement in patient symptomatology or objective measures compared with placebo. These studies are greatly limited by the use of empiric, not culture-directed, antibiotics. Currently, both these approaches remain investigatory and are not yet recommended based on current clinical evidence.

Corticosteroids

In broad strokes, chronic rhinosinusitis is currently categorized based on the presence or absence of polyposis.[1] Nasal polyposis and its predominantly eosinophilic inflammation have profound implications on the medical management of chronic rhinosinusitis – especially because it pertains to corticosteroids. As in acute rhinosinusitis, intranasal corticosteroids have proved useful for the treatment of chronic rhinosinusitis with or without polyposis, leading to decreased mucosal edema and significant symptomatic relief.[17] Furthermore, they have proved relatively safe for long-term treatment of chronic sinusitis as well as any underlying allergic rhinitis. In contrast to the treatment of acute frontal sinusitis, oral corticosteroid therapy has been shown to play a crucial role for the treatment of chronic frontal sinusitis, particularly in cases of chronic sinusitis with polyposis. Systemic corticosteroids have been shown to produce significant decrease in polyp burden as well as improved scores on sinonasal quality-of-life measures and thus have been used as a sort of medical polypectomy.[18] As discussed previously, however, prescribers must always take into account and inform patients of the potential side effects of systemic corticosteroids, particularly for prolonged courses that may be required for treatment of chronic rhinosinusitis with polyps.

The success of corticosteroids in chronic sinusitis have sparked interest in more-aggressive topical corticosteroid regimens in hopes of achieving the same beneficial clinical impact of systemic administration while maintaining the safety profile of topical administration. One particularly promising approach is the use of high-dose intranasal budesonide irrigations. In the context of chronic rhinosinusitis with polyposis, budesonide aqueous nasal solutions have been demonstrated to lead to reduced polyp burden and improved symptom scores, suggesting that they may be helpful in the context of chronic frontal sinusitis secondary to nasal polyposis. Additionally, although budesonide may have more systemic absorption compared with topical nasal steroid sprays, it has not been shown to cause any significant derangement of the hypothalamic-pituitary axis.[19] According to the most current clinical practice guidelines, however, their use is not yet recommended, because more rigorous investigation is still needed.

Antifungals

The role of antifungals in the medical management of chronic rhinosinusitis is one that has been hotly debated. Early research into the pathophysiology of chronic rhinosinusitis identified eosinophilic predominance, which, in conjunction with the presence of fungi on cultures of surgical specimens, led to the theory that chronic rhinosinusitis is the result of a deranged immunologic response to common environmental fungi.[20] Systemic and topical antifungals were suggested as a possible pharmacotherapy that could hold promise for the treatment of chronic rhinosinusitis. Despite initial promise, however, subsequent well-designed studies did not demonstrate the anticipated clinical benefit of antifungals in chronic sinusitis.[1] As such, antifungals are not recommended for the medical management of chronic frontal sinusitis.

Allergy Testing and Immunotherapy

Current understanding of chronic rhinosinusitis suggests that it is the result of local factors leading to mucosal edema, impaired sinus drainage, and bacterial overgrowth, all of which may contribute to sinonasal inflammation. Therefore, any discussion of medical management of chronic frontal sinusitis is incomplete without identification of these local factors and implementation of adjuvant therapies aimed at addressing them. For those patients with a clinical picture suggestive of allergic rhinitis, allergy testing may prove a useful diagnostic effort. Initiation of allergy immunotherapy is a powerful adjuvant that can alleviate mucosal inflammation and thus improve sinus ventilation and drainage. Allergy testing and immunotherapy have not demonstrated sufficient clinical benefit to warrant use in acute bacterial rhinosinusitis.[21]

Adjuvants

Finally, as with acute frontal sinusitis, the use of over-the-counter adjuvant therapies has also been shown useful. Nasal saline is an effective tool in the removal of tenacious mucus and secretions; however, consideration should be given to the mechanism of delivery. Although both saline irrigations and sprays are effective tools, irrigations have been shown more effective in the context of chronic sinusitis.[22] Furthermore, as in acute frontal sinusitis, topical nasal decongestants have been shown to decrease mucosal edema and thus improve sinus drainage and ventilation.

FUNGAL DISEASES OF THE FRONTAL SINUS
Allergic Fungal Sinusitis

Allergic fungal sinusitis is a common clinical entity defined by an allergic response to ubiquitous fungi and diagnosed based on several diagnostic criteria proposed by Bent and Kuhn.[23] Although this disease most commonly affects the maxillary sinus, it can also affect the frontal sinus. The management of allergic fungal sinusitis of the frontal sinuses is largely surgical, aimed at opening the affected sinus to drain the characteristic thick, eosinophilic mucin and improving sinus drainage. Medical comanagement does, however, play an important role.[24] Topical and systemic corticosteroids can be used to blunt the abnormal immunologic response found in allergic fungal sinusitis and thus are useful adjuvants, especially in the perioperative period. Additionally, allergy immunotherapy aimed at identifying and desensitizing the response to the causative organism has also shown promise. Although topical or systemic antifungals would intuitively play a role in allergic fungal sinusitis, neither has demonstrated any significant benefit in radiographic disease severity or symptomatology, thus reflecting the still incomplete understanding of the disease process itself.[25,26]

Fungal Ball

Discussion of the medical management of fungal infections of the frontal sinuses is not complete without discussion of its limitations. Fungal ball, or mycetoma, is a localized noninvasive colonization of fungus. Occurring most commonly in the maxillary sinus, it can also occur in the frontal sinus and is notoriously unresponsive to either antifungals or corticosteroids. Effective management of frontal sinus fungus balls requires surgical débridement and attempts at medical management should be avoided, given that they are ill advised and likely only delay definitive surgical intervention.[27]

Invasive Fungal Sinusitis

Whereas the aforementioned disease processes involve noninvasive fungal infections of the frontal sinuses, invasive fungal sinusitis differs fundamentally. Invasive fungal sinusitis, typically afflicting those with underlying immunocompromise, is a rare disease entity that can affect the frontal sinuses. Treatment of invasive fungal sinusitis is centered on aggressive surgical débridement to decrease pathogen load as well as initiation of systemic antifungals.[24] Despite surgical and medical comanagement, morbidity and mortality are high and frontal sinus involvement portends a poor prognosis given its close proximity to intracranial and orbital contents.

COMPLEMENTARY AND ALTERNATIVE THERAPIES

Complementary and alternative therapy is a term used to define a varied class of therapies outside the realm of traditional medical management. Although the purported benefits of these alternative therapies remain largely nebulous given a lack of in-depth research, it is of utmost importance to properly council patients regarding their use. In the context of medical management of frontal sinusitis there is no definitive benefit to alternative therapies, whether in the form of nutritional herbal supplements or traditional medicines.[28] Discussing the potential risks and benefits of these therapies and engaging in shared decision making with patients are crucial, however, for the maintenance of a strong patient-physician relationship and early identification of any potential adverse effects.

FUTURE DIRECTIONS

Ultimately no discussion of the medical management of frontal sinusitis would be complete without consideration of breakthroughs on the horizon. One technology that holds significant promise is the use of bioabsorbable steroid-eluting implants for maintenance of frontal sinus ostial patency after endoscopic sinus surgery. This same technology has already been shown to hold significant benefit when used in postoperative ethmoid cavities—reducing adhesions, middle turbinate lateralization, and polypoid change.[29] Studies are currently under way to evaluate the application of this same technology in maintenance of frontal sinus ostial patency after frontal sinusotomy. If successful, this type of localized drug delivery could be a powerful adjuvant in the management of frontal sinusitis.

REFERENCES

1. Meltzer EO, Hamilos DL, Hadley JA, et al. Rhinosinusitis: establishing definitions for clinical research and patient care. Otolaryngol Head Neck Surg 2004; 131(Suppl 6):S1–62.
2. Rosenfeld RM, Piccirillo JF, Chandrasekhar SS, et al. Clinical practice guideline: adult sinusitis. Otolaryngol Head Neck Surg 2015;152(S2):s1–39.
3. Lang E, Curran A, Patil N, et al. Intracranial complications of acute frontal sinusitis. Clin Otolaryngol Allied Sci 2001;26(6):452–7.
4. Brook I. Bacteriology of acute and chronic frontal sinusitis. Arch Otolaryngol Head Neck Surg 2002;128:583–5.
5. Brook I. Bacteriology of chronic maxillary sinusitis in adults. Ann Otol Rhinol Laryngol 1989;98:426–8.
6. Sinus and Allergy Health Partnership (SAHP). Antimicrobial treatment guidelines for acute bacterial rhinosinusitis. Otolaryngol Head Neck Surg 2004;130:1–45.
7. Harrison CJ, Woods C, Stout G, et al. Susceptibilities of Haemophilus influenzae, Streptococcus pneumoniae, including serotype 19A, and Moraxella catarrhalis paediatric isolates from 2005 to 2007 to commonly used antibiotics. J Antimicrob Chemother 2009;63:511–9.
8. Caenan M, Hamels K, Deron P, et al. Comparison of decongestive capacity of xylometazoline and pseudoephedrine with rhinomanometry and MRI. Rhinology 2005;43:205–9.
9. Keojampa BK, Nguyen MH, Ryan MW. Effects of buffered saline solution on nasal mucociliary clearance and nasal airway patency. Otolaryngol Head Neck Surg 2004;131:679–82.
10. Venekamp RP, Thompson MJ, Rovers MM. Systemic corticosteroid therapy for acute sinusitis. JAMA 2015;313(12):1258–9.
11. Zalmanovici A, Yaphe J. Intranasal steroids for acute sinusitis. Cochrane Database Syst Rev 2013;(2):CD005149.
12. Venekamp RP, Thompson MJ, Hayward G, et al. Systemic corticosteroids for acute sinusitis. Cochrane Database Syst Rev 2014;(3):CD008115.
13. Schlosser RJ, London SD, Gwaltney JM Jr, et al. Microbiology of chronic frontal sinusitis. Laryngoscope 2001;111:1330–2.
14. Thanasumpun T, Bara PS. Endoscopically-derived bacterial cultures in chronic rhinosinusitis: A systematic review. Am J Otolaryngol 2015;36(5):686–91.
15. Manarey CR, Anand VK, Huang C. Incidence of methicillin-resistant Staphylococcus aureus causing chronic rhinosinusitis. Laryngoscope 2004;114(5):939–41.
16. Soler ZM, Smith TL. What is the role of long-term macrolide therapy in the treatment of recalcitrant chronic rhinosinusitis? Laryngoscope 2009;119(9):1–2.
17. Vining EM. Evolution of medical management of chronic rhinosinusitis. Ann Otol Rhinol Laryngol Suppl 2006;196:54–60.
18. Patiar S, Reece P. Oral steroids for nasal polyps. Cochrane Database Syst Rev 2007;(1):CD005232.
19. Wei CC, Adappa ND, Cohen NA. Use of topical nasal therapies in the management of chronic Rhinosinusitis. Laryngoscope 2013;123(10):2347–59.
20. Sasama J, Sherris DA, Shin SH, et al. New paradigm for the roles of fungi and eosinophils in chronic rhinosinusitis. Curr Opin Otolaryngol Head Neck Surg 2005;13(1):2–8.
21. Frerichs KA, Nigten G, Romeijn K. Inconclusive evidence for allergic rhinitis to predict a prolonged or chronic course of acute rhinosinusitis. Otolaryngol Head Neck Surg 2014;150:22–7.

22. Harvey R, Hannan SA, Badia L, et al. Nasal saline irrigations for the symptoms of chronic rhinosinusitis. Cochrane Database Syst Rev 2007;(3):CD006394.

23. Bent JP 3rd, Kuhn FA. Diagnosis of allergic fungal sinusitis. Otolaryngol Head Neck Surg 1994;111(5):580–8.

24. Marple BF. Allergic fungal rhinosinusitis: current theories and management strategies. Laryngoscope 2001;111(6):1006–19.

25. Kennedy DW, Kuhn FA, Hamilos DL, et al. Treatment of chronic rhinosinusitis with high-dose oral terbinafine: a double blind, placebo-controlled study. Laryngoscope 2005;115(10):1793–9.

26. Stankiewicz JA, Musgrave BK, Scianna JM. Nasal amphotericin irrigation in chronic rhinosinusitis. Curr Opin Otolaryngol Head Neck Surg 2008;16(1):44–6.

27. Popko M, Broglie MA, Holzmann D. Isolated fungus ball mimicking mucocele or frontal sinus tumour: a diagnostic pitfall. J Laryngol Otol 2010;124:1111–5.

28. Roehm CE, Tessema B, Brown SM. The role of alternative medicine in rhinology. Facial Plast Surg Clin North Am 2012;20(1):73–81.

29. Marple BF, Smith TL, Han JK, et al. Advance II: a prospective, randomized study assessing safety and efficacy of bioabsorbable steroid-releasing sinus implants. Otolaryngol Head Neck Surg 2012;146:1004–11.

Anatomic Considerations in Frontal Sinus Surgery

Adam J. Folbe, MD[a,b,*], Peter F. Svider, MD[c], Jean Anderson Eloy, MD[d,e,f,g]

KEYWORDS

- Frontal sinus surgery • Frontal sinus outflow tract • Frontal sinusitis • Agger nasi cell
- Endoscopic sinus surgery • Frontal sinusotomy

KEY POINTS

- The three-dimensional anatomy of the frontal sinus and its outflow tract is complex and demonstrates a great degree of variability among patients. Consequently, careful examination of preoperative computed tomography and familiarity with each individual's anatomy are crucial for performance of a safe and successful surgical intervention.
- Familiarity with the presence and location of the anterior ethmoid artery, uncinate bone, agger nasi cells, suprabullar cells, and frontal cells is critical before frontal sinus surgery; furthermore, knowledge of the extent of pneumatization and development of each frontal sinus is mandatory.
- Visualization of the frontal sinus recess through a sagittal view allows for appreciation of the agger nasi cell (anteriorly), suprabullar cells (posteriorly), vertical lamella of the middle turbinate (medially), fovea ethmoidalis (posteriorly), lateral lamella (posteromedially), and the orbit (laterally).
- For patients in whom the agger nasi cell comprises a large portion of the frontal recess, endoscopic visualization of this cell can be confused with the frontal recess itself. The use of image guidance, switching to a 70° endoscope, and palpation of the middle turbinate can assist in making this distinction.

Continued

Financial Disclosures: None.

Conflicts of Interest: None.

[a] Rhinology and Sinus Surgery, Department of Otolaryngology–Head and Neck Surgery, Wayne State University School of Medicine, St. Antoine, Detroit, MI 48201, USA; [b] Department of Neurosurgery, Wayne State University School of Medicine, St. Antoine, Detroit, MI 48201, USA; [c] Department of Otolaryngology–Head and Neck Surgery, Wayne State University School of Medicine, St. Antoine, Detroit, MI 48201, USA; [d] Department of Otolaryngology–Head and Neck Surgery, Rutgers New Jersey Medical School, Newark, NJ, USA; [e] Center for Skull Base and Pituitary Surgery, Rutgers New Jersey Medical School, Newark, NJ, USA; [f] Department of Neurological Surgery, Rutgers New Jersey Medical School, Newark, NJ, USA; [g] Department of Ophthalmology and Visual Science, Rutgers New Jersey Medical School, Newark, NJ, USA

* Corresponding author. Rhinology and Sinus Surgery, Department of Otolaryngology–Head and Neck Surgery, Wayne State University School of Medicine, Detroit, MI

E-mail address: afolbe@gmail.com

Otolaryngol Clin N Am 49 (2016) 935–943

http://dx.doi.org/10.1016/j.otc.2016.03.017

0030-6665/16/$ – see front matter © 2016 Elsevier Inc. All rights reserved.

oto.theclinics.com

Continued

- External procedures, including trephination and osteoplastic flap with obliteration, harbor potential morbidities including scarring, persistent pain, and the risk of intracranial/orbital injuries; nonetheless, these procedures may have utility in certain situations, including inaccessible lateral disease, patients with severe scarring, and other anatomic variations.

Abbreviations
BCD   Balloon catheter dilation
CT   Computed tomography

Comprehension of the complex anatomic variants comprising the frontal sinus outflow tract is essential for successful surgical intervention. Similar to consideration of the other paranasal sinuses, familiarity with the surrounding anatomy in both virgin and revision cases is critical, because deviation from sound technique has the potential to result in a variety of sequelae ranging from recurrent disease to catastrophic intracranial and orbital injury. Furthermore, the frontal sinus outflow tract is typically a tight space where even a small amount of mucosal disruption can lead to the failure of any intervention. Consequently, a detailed understanding of the surgical anatomy is paramount.

Frontal sinus surgical intervention has evolved since the era of trephination and obliteration. Nonetheless, although rarely performed, these open procedures still arguably have a role in the otolaryngologist's surgical repertoire.[1] Hence, a thorough understanding of both endoscopic visualization and anatomic considerations relating to external techniques may be valuable for the practicing otolaryngologist. This review aims to cover the key anatomy encountered, further illustrating these concepts through a description of several advanced dissection techniques.

SURGICAL PLANNING

As in any operative procedure, appropriate preoperative assessment and exhausting all nonsurgical options as appropriate are critical. Comprehensively reviewing medical management of frontal sinus disease as well as indications and contraindications for surgical intervention is beyond the scope of this review, but its importance cannot be overemphasized. With regard to frontal sinus anatomical considerations, close examination of preoperative imaging is mandatory. Nowadays, this almost exclusively encompasses computed tomography (CT), preferably involving fine cuts with axial, coronal, and sagittal views. Key structures to examine include the location of the anterior ethmoid artery (**Fig. 1**), the presence and amount of suprabullar cells (**Fig. 2**), the presence of the agger nasi cell (and its degree of pneumatization) (see **Fig. 2**; **Fig. 3**), the depth and pneumatization of the frontal sinuses, the uncinate bone attachment, and middle turbinate anatomy.[2] Each of these landmarks is discussed in further detail later. Visualization of the frontal sinus recess through a sagittal view allows for appreciation of its basic anatomic features (see **Fig. 2**). In relation to the frontal recess, the agger nasi cell is often present anteriorly, suprabullar cells posteriorly, fovea ethmoidalis posteriorly (see **Fig. 2**), the middle turbinate (vertical lamella) medially (see **Fig. 1**), lateral lamella posteromedially, and the orbit laterally.[1–4]

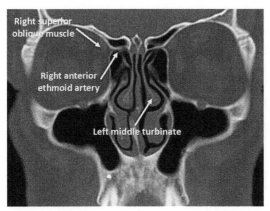

Fig. 1. Coronal CT scan illustrating location of the right anterior ethmoid artery, adjacent to the right superior oblique muscle.

THE UNCINATE PROCESS

The attachment of the uncinate process impacts the drainage of the frontal sinus. In the most common configuration, the uncinate process attaches to the medial orbital wall, resulting in a drainage pattern medial to the uncinate and directly into the middle meatus.[3] In the minority of cases that involve uncinate attachment to the middle turbinate or skull base, drainage occurs lateral to the uncinate. Preoperative evaluation of imaging and familiarity with the uncinate attachment are helpful knowledge for the surgeon.

AGGER NASI CELLS

The presence and extent of agger nasi cell development are among the most important factors with which to be familiar before operating on a patient for frontal sinus disease. Being the most anterior ethmoid air cell, it represents the anterior border of the frontal recess (see **Figs. 2** and **3**), and its size and pneumatization can have a significant impact on frontal sinus outflow in combination with mucosal integrity and other

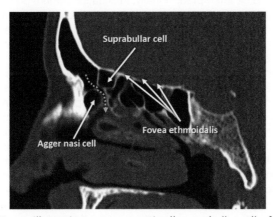

Fig. 2. Sagittal CT scan illustrating an agger nasi cell, suprabullar cells, fovea ethmoidalis, and frontal sinus outflow tract (*arrow*).

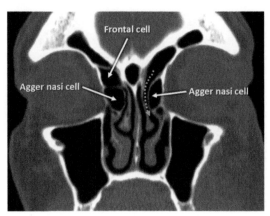

Fig. 3. Coronal CT scan illustrating bilateral agger nasi cells, a right type I frontal cell, and left frontal sinus outflow tract (*arrow*).

immunologic factors. Preoperative imaging should be examined for these factors. Although originally thought to have a lower prevalence, improvements in CT revealed that this cell is present in nearly all patients.[5,6] It can be found on a coronal scan associated with the origin of the middle turbinate.[4] As described later, removing the posterior wall of this cell is instrumental for facilitating frontal sinus drainage in advanced frontal sinusotomy. On endoscopic view, the agger nasi cell manifests as a "bulge" or "mound" anterior to the origin of the middle turbinate on the lateral nasal wall.[5]

In patients with larger agger nasi cells comprising a significant portion of the frontal recess, this cell can be confused with the frontal sinus recess itself. Several strategies can be used if there is intraoperative uncertainty regarding whether one is in the frontal sinus recess. The surgeon can gently palpate the posterior wall of what is thought to be the frontal sinus recess as well as the middle turbinate with a probe. If a completely different bony wall is found, the surgeon can gently remove this wall. Another method that may assist in determining whether one is in the frontal sinus recess or an agger nasi cell is switching endoscopes. Switching to a 70° camera and visualizing the entire frontal recess should be attempted.[5] Finally, in situations where preoperative imaging indicates complicated frontal sinus recess anatomy, including significant agger nasi cells, image guidance may play a role,[7] although the investigators stress that this tool should be used as an adjunct in surgery rather than be relied on.

The importance of understanding whether one's probes and instruments are located in the frontal sinus recess versus an agger nasi cell cannot be emphasized enough. A recent analysis of chronic rhinosinusitis patients with endoscopic sinus surgery failures noted that retained agger nasi cells were present in the majority (73.1%), likely contributing to persistent symptoms.[8] If one mistakenly thinks they are not in an agger nasi cell and that the frontal sinus recess is not obstructed, then frontal sinus obstruction may obviously remain postoperatively. Furthermore, leaving a portion of the agger nasi cell may facilitate further outflow tract scarring, as the remnants may adhere to the posterior wall of the frontal sinus recess.[5] Finally, with newer technologies, such as balloon catheter dilation (BCD), situations may occur where a balloon is deployed into an agger nasi cell (rather than the frontal recess), and resultant dilation may cause frontal sinus recess obstruction worse than what was initially present, necessitating a more difficult revision procedure down the road.

ANTERIOR ETHMOID ARTERY

Running across the fovea ethmoidalis, the anterior ethmoid artery (see **Fig. 1**) is approximately 1 cm behind the frontal sinus infundibulum or within 1.5 to 2.5 cm of the middle turbinate's anterior attachment.[2,9] When present, extracranial anterior ethmoid artery can be identified on preoperative CT and is often next to the superior oblique muscle (see **Fig. 1**).[10] It is important to be cognizant of its location, because breaching this structure can result in considerable hemorrhage, resultantly poor visualization, and even retraction into the orbit causing orbital hemorrhage.[10–14]

FRONTAL SINUS CELLS

There are several types of frontal cells, initially defined by Bent and Kuhn, that are important to identify on preoperative imaging.[1,15–17] Retrospective reviews note that approximately 20% of individuals have frontal cells on CT.[16] In patients with symptoms, these may need to be removed to facilitate drainage and address disease. Type I frontal cells (see **Fig. 2**) do not involve the sinus itself, but are single cells located above the agger nasi cell that occlude the frontal recess. They are generally the most prevalent and are thought to have a significant association with frontal sinus mucosal thickening.[15] Type II cells involve multiple cells above the agger nasi interfering with drainage, although by definition these do not extend into the actual frontal sinus. A type III frontal cell does extend into the frontal sinus superiorly from the agger nasi, while a type IV cell is a solitary cell in the frontal sinus.

SUPRABULLAR CELLS

Although the previously discussed agger nasi and frontal sinus cells are located in the anterior border of the frontal sinus recess, the suprabullar cells represent an important component of the posterior frontal sinus recess (see **Fig. 2**). Noting the presence and extent of suprabullar cells on preoperative imaging provides valuable information to the frontal sinus surgeon regarding how close one is to the skull base. Furthermore, these posterior cells, including suprabullar, frontal bullar, and supraorbital ethmoid cells (**Fig. 4**), may have a higher association with chronic frontal sinusitis, increasing the importance of addressing them adequately.[18] When addressing the suprabullar cells, the surgeon should take care to direct dissection in an anterior-inferior trajectory

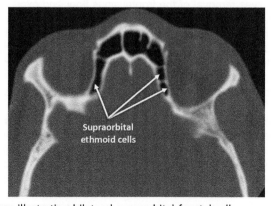

Fig. 4. Axial CT scan illustrating bilateral supraorbital frontal cells.

in order to prevent disruption of the skull base, particularly in the neighborhood of the anterior ethmoid artery.[2]

APPLIED SURGICAL ANATOMY: ENDOSCOPIC FRONTAL SINUSOTOMY

Although the goals of this article include detailing surgically relevant anatomy rather than surgical technique, the Draf approaches stress many of the anatomic principles described earlier and demonstrate the importance of familiarity with endoscopic anatomy. A thorough understanding of these approaches reinforces surgical anatomic principles and highlights potential pitfalls. In later discussion, the authors detail the basic objectives of endoscopic frontal sinusotomy, because they share the common goal of removing obstacles to frontal sinus outflow.

After failed adequate nonsurgical management options, frontal sinus drainage can oftentimes be optimized by performing an adequate ethmoidectomy. Ethmoidectomy involves addressing any suprabullar cells when present as well as removal of the ethmoid bulla cell. Performance of this approach, without any instrumentation involving the frontal sinus recess mucosa, is a Draf I procedure.[1,19,20] In addition, a Draf I frontal sinusotomy is generally understood to include the outflow tract of the frontal recess and dissection of the posterior wall of the agger nasi cell. This dissection is directed inferiorly, ensuring that is it not toward the skull base, and ultimately results in a widened frontal recess.[1] A BCD is one way to complete at Draf I procedure.

The Draf IIa endoscopic frontal sinusotomy, oftentimes performed for persistent disease after a Draf I procedure, directly involves the frontal recess and results in an open pathway from the medial orbital wall to the middle turbinate.[1,20] In addition to removal of the agger nasi cell as previously described, other cells involving the frontal recess are addressed (type I–IV frontal cells), and the roof of the most superior suprabullar cell is removed.[1,2] All disease and cells from the frontal sinus laterally to the middle turbinate medially are removed. When instruments are directed into the frontal sinus recess, it is of utmost importance to avoid directing instrumentation too far medially, because this may violate the thin lateral lamella of the cribriform region, potentially resulting in cerebrospinal fluid leak, and other possible intracranial complications. After these cells have been removed, transillumination can be performed to ensure one is in the frontal sinus.[1]

An extended frontal sinusotomy may be appropriate in several situations involving severe disease, including in patients with excessive scarring and polyposis occluding frontal sinus outflow. The Draf IIb approach addresses the same structures as in a Draf IIa procedure, involves removal of the frontal sinus floor and excision of the anterior portion of the middle turbinate.[1,19,20] To avoid compromising the skull base, it is important to only remove the turbinate in a coronal plane anterior to the posterior frontal sinus table.[21] Ultimately, a Draf IIb results in a fully open outflow tract from the lamina papyracea laterally to the nasal septum medially. Although controversial, some investigators feel the Draf IIb procedure results in a high chance of scarring, recommending avoidance of this approach in patients with inflammatory disease like chronic rhinosinusitis.[20,22,23]

Also known as a modified Lothrop approach, the Draf III approach involves the same steps as a Draf IIb bilaterally in addition to removal of the intersinus septum. Furthermore, removal of a portion of the anterosuperior nasal septum is performed, starting at the frontal sinus ostium and continuing 1 to 2 cm anteriorly. This procedure results in a unified frontal sinus outflow tract. Indications for a Draf III include disease in the lateral recess that cannot be accessed using more conservative approaches as well as patients harboring persistent disease and symptoms following a Draf II procedure.[1]

SURGICAL ANATOMY AND EXTERNAL APPROACHES

With the advent of advanced endoscopic techniques, there are some who have questioned whether a role remains for external approaches to the frontal sinus. These open procedures, including trephination and osteoplastic flap obliteration, harbor considerable potential morbidities (including orbital and intracranial intrusion) and may impact cosmesis. Visible scarring is certainly one consideration, whereas an external approach may result in considerably more pain for many patients.[24] Nonetheless, some suggest these procedures may be used as a primary strategy or adjunct in special situations, and modifications have been proposed over the years to minimize deleterious sequelae.[25–28] Specific indications for using these techniques include very lateral disease not accessible via a purely endoscopic approach, certain types of tumors, as well as severe scarring and other anatomic variations that may make endoscopic intervention fraught with hazard.

Whether performing osteoplastic flap with or without obliteration, several anatomic considerations are essential when planning frontal sinus trephination. Image guidance may be a useful adjunct for finding the midline of the floor of the sinus, because this is where the frontal sinus is the largest anteroposterior diameter, minimizing chances of breaching the posterior table.[26] Osteoplastic flap obliteration, which may also involve trephination or the use of endoscopes as an adjunct, may be used in repair of frontal sinus fractures, persistent disease, tumors, and mucoceles. In addition to CT imaging, external frontal sinus procedures including the osteoplastic flap are among the few situations where plain film radiographs may still play a role.[29] A 6-foot Caldwell view is used as a template directing the placement of bone cuts. It is important to ensure that this template is accurate (ie, taken from an accurate distance), because the use of an inaccurate template may result in catastrophic injuries from sawing and drilling toward orbital and intracranial structures.[30] Knowledge of the facial nerve's frontal branch is paramount; staying immediately deep to the superficial temporal fascia will avoid this branch.[27,31] After getting down to the superior orbital rim, at this point a radiograph template can be used in order to mark the borders of the frontal sinus, and either trephination or use of an endoscope intranasally can be used to confirm the frontal sinus location via transillumination. After elevating the periosteum, the bone cuts can be performed and all frontal sinus mucosa is removed. Harvested fat is placed and the bone flap is covered over this, followed by closure.[30,32,33] Failure to remove all of the frontal sinus mucosa can lead to mucocele formation down the road.

IMAGE GUIDANCE IN FRONTAL SINUS SURGERY

Although its routine use is not necessary, intraoperative image guidance systems may play a helpful role in frontal sinus surgical intervention. This modality may be useful in cases involving revision procedures and complicated outflow anatomic variants and can also be useful as an adjunct in external approaches.[34] Regardless, it is certainly not a substitute for familiarity with endoscopic and external frontal sinus anatomy, and there is no consensus demonstrating an increase in efficacy, decrease in complications, or decrease in medicolegal liability through its use.[10,34–37]

SUMMARY

An understanding of the complicated 3-dimensional anatomy of the frontal sinus and its outflow tract is critical for safe and successful frontal sinus surgery. Although novel technologies such as intraoperative surgical navigation may be a valuable adjunct, familiarity with the relevant anatomy is mandatory for minimizing recurrence and serious adverse events. Gathered from careful preoperative review of imaging and appropriate endoscopic technique, awareness of the anterior ethmoid artery, insertion and anatomy of the uncinate process, the extent of the agger nasi cell development, and the presence of suprabullar and frontal sinus cells all influence surgical planning. Although application of these principles to endoscopic techniques is essential, knowledge of external techniques may be a valuable addition to the sinus surgeon's armamentarium in certain situations.

REFERENCES

1. Folbe AJ, Svider PF, Eloy JA. Advances in endoscopic frontal sinus surgery. Operat Tech Otolaryngol Head Neck Surg 2014;25:180–6.
2. Casiano RR, Herzallah IR, Anstead A, et al. Basic endoscopic sinonasal dissection. In: Casiano RR, editor. Endoscopic sinonasal dissection guide. New York: Thieme; 2012. p. 19–58.
3. Daniels DL, Mafee MF, Smith MM, et al. The frontal sinus drainage pathway and related structures. AJNR Am J Neuroradiol 2003;24:1618–27.
4. Wormald PJ. Three-dimensional building block approach to understanding the anatomy of the frontal recess and frontal sinus. Otolaryngol Head Neck Surg 2006;17:2–5.
5. Kuhn FA, Bolger WE, Tisdal RG. The agger nasi cell in frontal recess obstruction: an anatomic, radiologic and clinical correlation. Otolaryngol Head Neck Surg 1991;2:226–31.
6. Bolger WE, Butzin CA, Parsons DS. Paranasal sinus bony anatomic variations and mucosal abnormalities: CT analysis for endoscopic sinus surgery. Laryngoscope 1991;101:56–64.
7. Chiu AG, Vaughan WC. Revision endoscopic frontal sinus surgery with surgical navigation. Otolaryngol Head Neck Surg 2004;130:312–8.
8. Valdes CJ, Bogado M, Samaha M. Causes of failure in endoscopic frontal sinus surgery in chronic rhinosinusitis patients. Int Forum Allergy Rhinol 2014;4:502–6.
9. Lee WC, Ming Ku PK, van Hasselt CA. New guidelines for endoscopic localization of the anterior ethmoidal artery: a cadaveric study. Laryngoscope 2000; 110:1173–8.
10. Svider PF, Baredes S, Eloy JA. Pitfalls in sinus surgery: an overview of complications. Otolaryngol Clin North Am 2015;48(5):725–37.
11. Dutton JJ. Orbital complications of paranasal sinus surgery. Ophthal Plast Reconstr Surg 1986;2:119–27.
12. Han JK, Higgins TS. Management of orbital complications in endoscopic sinus surgery. Curr Opin Otolaryngol Head Neck Surg 2010;18:32–6.
13. Stankiewicz JA, Chow JM. Two faces of orbital hematoma in intranasal (endoscopic) sinus surgery. Otolaryngol Head Neck Surg 1999;120:841–7.
14. Eloy JA, Svider PF, Setzen M. Clinical pearls in endoscopic sinus surgery: key steps in preventing and dealing with complications. Am J Otolaryngol 2014;35: 324–8.
15. Langille M, Walters E, Dziegielewski PT, et al. Frontal sinus cells: identification, prevalence, and association with frontal sinus mucosal thickening. Am J Rhinol Allergy 2012;26:e107–10.
16. Meyer TK, Kocak M, Smith MM, et al. Coronal computed tomography analysis of frontal cells. Am J Rhinol 2003;17:163–8.
17. Tuncyurek O, Songu M, Adibelli ZH, et al. Frontal infundibular cells: pathway to the frontal sinus. Ear Nose Throat J 2012;91:E29–32.

18. Lien CF, Weng HH, Chang YC, et al. Computed tomographic analysis of frontal recess anatomy and its effect on the development of frontal sinusitis. Laryngoscope 2010;120:2521–7.

19. Draf W, Weber R, Keerl R, et al. Current aspects of frontal sinus surgery. I: endonasal frontal sinus drainage in inflammatory diseases of the paranasal sinuses. HNO 1995;43:352–7 [Article in German].

20. Weber R, Draf W, Kratzsch B, et al. Modern concepts of frontal sinus surgery. Laryngoscope 2001;111:137–46.

21. Eloy JA, Liu JK, Choudhry OJ, et al. Modified subtotal Lothrop procedure for extended frontal sinus and anterior skull base access: a cadaveric feasibility study with clinical correlates. J Neurol Surg B Skull Base 2013;74:130–5.

22. Samaha M, Cosenza MJ, Metson R. Endoscopic frontal sinus drillout in 100 patients. Arch Otolaryngol Head Neck Surg 2003;129:854–8.

23. Fokkens WJ, Jones NS. Management of the frontal sinus. In: Flint PW, Haughey BH, Lund VJ, et al, editors. Cummings otolaryngology. 6th edition. New York: Elsevier; 2015. p. 790–802.

24. Hardy JM, Montgomery WW. Osteoplastic frontal sinusotomy: an analysis of 250 operations. Ann Otol Rhinol Laryngol 1976;85:523–32.

25. Batra PS, Citardi MJ, Lanza DC. Combined endoscopic trephination and endoscopic frontal sinusotomy for management of complex frontal sinus pathology. Am J Rhinol 2005;19:435–41.

26. Lee AS, Schaitkin BM, Gillman GS. Evaluating the safety of frontal sinus trephination. Laryngoscope 2010;120:639–42.

27. Patel AB, Cain RB, Lal D. Contemporary applications of frontal sinus trephination: a systematic review of the literature. Laryngoscope 2015;125(9):2046–53.

28. Seiberling K, Jardeleza C, Wormald PJ. Minitrephination of the frontal sinus: indications and uses in today's era of sinus surgery. Am J Rhinol Allergy 2009;23:229–31.

29. Fung MK. Template for frontal osteoplastic flap. Laryngoscope 1986;96:578–9.

30. Maniglia AJ, Dodds BL. A safe technique for frontal sinus osteoplastic flap. Laryngoscope 1991;101:908–10.

31. Schneider JS, Day A, Clavena M, et al. Early practice: external sinus surgery and procedures and complications. Otolaryngol Clin North Am 2015;48(5):839–50.

32. Calcaterra TC, Strahan RW. Osteoplastic flap technique for disease of the frontal sinus. Surg Gynecol Obstet 1971;132:505–10.

33. Hahn S, Palmer JN, Purkey MT, et al. Indications for external frontal sinus procedures for inflammatory sinus disease. Am J Rhinol Allergy 2009;23:342–7.

34. Sindwani R, Metson R. Image-guided frontal sinus surgery. Otolaryngol Clin North Am 2005;38:461–71.

35. Eloy JA, Svider PF, D'Aguillo CM, et al. Image-guidance in endoscopic sinus surgery: is it associated with decreased medicolegal liability? Int Forum Allergy Rhinol 2013;3:980–5.

36. Eloy JA, Svider PF, Patel D, et al. Comparison of plaintiff and defendant expert witness qualification in malpractice litigation in otolaryngology. Otolaryngol Head Neck Surg 2013;148:764–9.

37. Ramakrishnan VR, Orlandi RR, Citardi MJ, et al. The use of image-guided surgery in endoscopic sinus surgery: an evidence-based review with recommendations. Int Forum Allergy Rhinol 2013;3:236–41.

Instrumentation in Frontal Sinus Surgery

Bobby A. Tajudeen, MD, Nithin D. Adappa, MD*

KEYWORDS

- Frontal recess • Frontal sinus surgery • Frontal sinus instrumentation
- Chronic sinusitis • Frontal sinusitis

KEY POINTS

- Sinus surgery failure occurs most commonly in the frontal recess and is largely attributable to surgical technique.
- Image guidance is an extremely helpful adjunct to complete frontal recess dissection even for the most experienced surgeons.
- Angled 45° and 70° endoscopes significantly improve visualization.
- The use of through-cutting hand instrumentation is critical for sound mucosal-sparing technique to minimize scar formation.
- Mucosal preservation is key, regardless of technique, to ensure frontal patency.

INTRODUCTION

The frontal recess comprises the intricate outflow tract of the frontal sinus and is bordered by the agger nasi cell anteriorly, the lamina papyracea laterally, the middle turbinate medially, and the bulla ethmoidalis posteriorly. In addition, there are many unique frontal cells that add to the level of surgical complexity. Dissection in the frontal recess proposes several challenges. These challenges include significant variable anatomy, challenging visualization, narrow caliber, proximity to vital structures including the skull base and orbit, and the need for advanced instrumentation. As such, sinus surgery failure occurs most commonly in the frontal recess.[1,2] Common findings at the time of revision frontal sinus surgery include edematous or hypertrophied mucosa, retained agger nasi cell, neo-osteogenesis within the frontal recess, lateral scarring of the middle turbinate, residual anterior ethmoid cells, and residual frontal cells.[1,2] With the exclusion of edema and neo-osteogenesis, the remaining causes are the direct result of surgical technique. Proper instrumentation is necessary for delicate mucosal-sparing surgical technique. Here, the authors

Department of Otorhinolaryngology–Head and Neck Surgery, The University of Pennsylvania, 3400 Spruce Street, 5 Ravdin, Philadelphia, PA 19104, USA
* Corresponding author.
E-mail address: Nithin.Adappa@Uphs.upenn.edu

Otolaryngol Clin N Am 49 (2016) 945–949
http://dx.doi.org/10.1016/j.otc.2016.03.018
0030-6665/16/$ – see front matter © 2016 Elsevier Inc. All rights reserved.

oto.theclinics.com

provide an overview of the current instrumentation and adjunctive technologies used commonly in complete frontal recess dissections.

IMAGE GUIDANCE

Image guidance can be a helpful adjunct to frontal recess dissection even for the most experienced surgeons. Aside from providing confirmation of complete frontal recess dissection, the image-guidance system planning station can be used preoperatively to study anatomic variants and help develop a plan for intraoperative dissection. The triplanar view that an image-guidance system provides gives the surgeon additional information to safely open the sinus. Individual preference and institutional availability should guide the decision to choose between electromagnetic or optical-based systems because both systems provide comparable accuracy in anatomic localization.[3,4]

ANGLED ENDOSCOPES

Proper visualization of is of utmost importance when performing frontal recess dissection. Although some describe frontal sinus surgery without angled endoscopes,[5] in general, a minimum of a 30°, and preferably a 70°, endoscope is needed for adequate visualization. Reverse or offset angled endoscopes are extremely helpful. Reverse endoscopes are designed with the light-post oriented superiorly, thus allowing for easier use of curved frontal sinus instruments because the light-post does obstruct access as it does with traditional endoscopes. Irrigating lens-cleaning sheaths can also be helpful to maintain a clear field.

HAND INSTRUMENTATION

The use of through-cutting hand instrumentation is critical for sound mucosal-sparing technique. A list of commonly used hand instrumentation in frontal recess dissection is listed in later discussion.

45° Mushroom Punch

The 45° mushroom (Karl Storz, Tuttlingen, Germany) punch is particularly useful to enlarge an existing opening circumferentially (**Fig. 1**). In addition, it is the only frontal

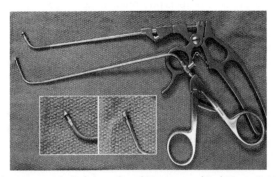

Fig. 1. A 45° mushroom punch (*left insert*) and Hosemann (Karl Storz, Tuttlingen, Germany) punch (*right insert*). The Hosemann punch is a 45° mushroom punch with greater cutting strength that allows for removal of thick bone, such as the floor of the frontal recess.

sinus hand instrument capable of removing horizontal partitions in an anterior to posterior direction in a through-cutting manner. This situation is commonly encountered in the posterior frontal recess. The Hosemann punch is similar to the 45° mushroom punch with much greater cutting strength (see **Fig. 1**). This instrument is best used for removal of osteitic bone of the frontal sinus floor.

Bachert Forceps

The Bachert forceps (Karl Storz, Tuttlingen, Germany) is an important tool for frontal recess dissection. This instrument resembles a 45° Kerrison punch that punches back to front (**Fig. 2**). The Bachert forceps is used to remove horizontal ledges, such as the caps of the agger nasi and frontal recess cells, in a back-to-front fashion.

Through-Cutting Giraffe Forceps

Through-cutting giraffe forceps (Karl Storz, Tuttlingen, Germany) come in side-to-side and front-to-back varieties at both 45° and 90° angles (**Fig. 3**). These instruments are helpful in removing vertically oriented partitions such as the posterior wall (front-to-back) and medial wall (side-to-side) of the agger nasi cell.

Non-Through-Cutting Frontal Giraffe Forceps

These forceps (Karl Storz, Tuttlingen, Germany) also come in side-to-side and front-to-back varieties at both 45° to 90° angles as well as different sizes (**Fig. 4**). They are useful to delicately pick out loose remnants of bone in a mucosal-sparing fashion. In addition, they can be used to pull out thick allergic fungal mucin or foreign bodies following prior trauma.

Frontal Probes and Curettes

A variety of supplementary frontal instruments including Kuhn probes and frontal curettes are also available (**Fig. 5**). Kuhn probes come in many versions and are generally ball-tipped, curved instruments that have extended length. They are very useful for high dissection of frontal recess cells. In addition, fine probes can be useful in avoiding trauma to delicate mucosa in a small-diameter frontal recess, where mucosal preservation is critical to ensure long-term patency.

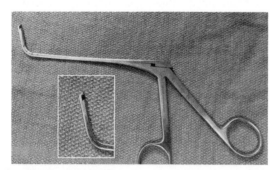

Fig. 2. A Bachert forceps. The Bachert forceps is used to remove horizontal ledges, such as the caps of the agger nasi and frontal recess cells, in a back-to-front fashion, and is considered the workhorse instrument for frontal recess dissection. This is available in several different sizes.

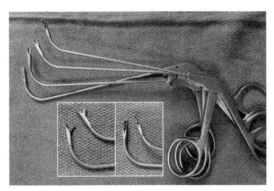

Fig. 3. Through-cutting giraffe forceps. These instruments come in side-to-side (*right insert*) and front-to-back (*left insert*) varieties at both 45° and 90° angles. These instruments allow for removal of vertically orientated partitions in a mucosal-sparing fashion.

POWERED INSTRUMENTATION

Powered instrumentation in frontal recess dissection includes powered microde-briders and drills. Microdebriders are available in a variety of sizes and angulations. The microdebrider should only be used to clean up free mucosal edges after the use of through-cutting hand instrumentation. Powered drills are also available in a variety of sizes and angles. The 70° diamond drill is safest (in the authors' opinion) and most useful. Drills are particularly useful when there is significant neo-osteogenesis or there is a prominent nasofrontal beak narrowing the frontal recess. It is also advised to reintroduce punches as bone is thinned with the drill to in-crease both speed and safety.

FUTURE DEVELOPMENTS

Additional adjuncts to frontal sinus dissection are continuously being developed. Perhaps most promising is the development of drug-eluting stents, which are postu-lated to improve postoperative frontal recess patency by acting as both a spacer and a drug-delivery system, minimizing mucosal edema and scarring. Three prospective, randomized, controlled trials and one meta-analysis have demonstrated the effective-ness of steroid-eluting stents when placed in the ethmoid sinus.[6–9] Smaller implants could prove useful in maintaining frontal recess patency; however, this has not been extensively studied.

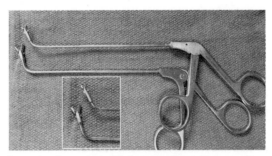

Fig. 4. Non-through-cutting frontal giraffe forceps. These instruments are also available in side-to-side and front-to-back varieties at both 45° and 90° angles.

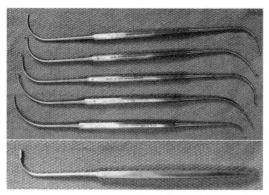

Fig. 5. Frontal probes (*top*) and a frontal curette (*bottom*) (Karl Storz, Tuttlingen, Germany). Frontal probes are useful in dissection of frontal recess cells that are located high in the frontal sinus.

SUMMARY

Frontal recess dissection is challenging and requires meticulous surgery. Proper instrumentation and visualization are imperative to enhance surgical precision, spare mucosa, and prevent the scarring and neo-osteogenesis that may cause surgical failures. A wide armamentarium of frontal sinus instrumentation is pivotal to performing safe frontal sinus surgery with long-term patency.

REFERENCES

1. Otto KJ, DelGaudio JM. Operative findings in the frontal recess at time of revision surgery. Am J Otolaryngol 2010;31(3):175–80.
2. Valdes CJ, Bogado M, Samaha M. Causes of failure in endoscopic frontal sinus surgery in chronic rhinosinusitis patients. Int Forum Allergy Rhinol 2014;4(6):502–6.
3. Metson R, Gliklich RE, Cosenza M. A comparison of image guidance systems for sinus surgery. Laryngoscope 1998;108(8 Pt 1):1164–70.
4. Wise SK, DelGaudio JM. Computer-aided surgery of the paranasal sinuses and skull base. Expert Rev Med Devices 2005;2(4):395–408.
5. Pletcher SD, Sindwani R, Metson R. The agger nasi punch-out procedure (POP): maximizing exposure of the frontal recess. Laryngoscope 2006;116(9):1710–2.
6. Forwith KD, Chandra RK, Yun PT, et al. ADVANCE: a multisite trial of bioabsorbable steroid-eluting sinus implants. Laryngoscope 2011;121(11):2473–80.
7. Han JK, Marple BF, Smith TL, et al. Effect of steroid-releasing sinus implants on postoperative medical and surgical interventions: an efficacy meta-analysis. Int Forum Allergy Rhinol 2012;2(4):271–9.
8. Marple BF, Smith TL, Han JK, et al. Advance II: a prospective, randomized study assessing safety and efficacy of bioabsorbable steroid-releasing sinus implants. Otolaryngol Head Neck Surg 2012;146(6):1004–11.
9. Murr AH, Smith TL, Hwang PH, et al. Safety and efficacy of a novel bioabsorbable, steroid-eluting sinus stent. Int Forum Allergy Rhinol 2011;1(1):23–32.

Preventing and Managing Complications in Frontal Sinus Surgery

Jean Anderson Eloy, MD[a,b,c,d],*, Peter F. Svider, MD[e],
Michael Setzen, MD[f,g]

KEYWORDS

- Frontal sinusitis • Balloon catheter dilation • Frontal sinusotomy
- Endoscopic sinus surgery • Endoscopic frontal sinus surgery • Orbital injury
- Cerebrospinal fluid leak • Frontal sinus outflow tract

KEY POINTS

- Preoperative management encompasses appropriate patient selection. With a few exceptions, patients undergoing surgical interventions for frontal sinusitis should have exhausted medical management options.
- The preoperative assessment also includes detailed evaluation of imaging for the integrity of the lamina papyracea, the presence of an extracranial anterior ethmoid artery, and anatomic variants impacting the frontal sinus outflow tract, such as accessory frontal sinus cells.
- A comprehensive informed consent includes frank discussion of the potential for significant adverse events, most notably anosmia, orbital complications, and cerebrospinal fluid rhinorrhea.

Continued

Financial Disclosures: None.
Conflicts of Interest: M. Setzen: Speaker's Bureau for Meda and Advisory Board for Merck and Lannett (not related to current subject).
[a] Department of Otolaryngology–Head and Neck Surgery, Rutgers New Jersey Medical School, 90 Bergen Street, Suite 8100, Newark, NJ 07103, USA; [b] Center for Skull Base and Pituitary Surgery, Neurological Institute of New Jersey, Rutgers New Jersey Medical School, Newark, NJ, USA; [c] Department of Neurological Surgery, Rutgers New Jersey Medical School, Newark, NJ, USA; [d] Department of Ophthalmology and Visual Science, Rutgers New Jersey Medical School, Newark, NJ, USA; [e] Department of Otolaryngology–Head and Neck Surgery, Wayne State University School of Medicine, Detroit, MI, USA; [f] Rhinology Section, North Shore University Hospital, Manhasset, NY, USA; [g] Department of Otolaryngology, New York University School of Medicine, New York, NY, USA
* Corresponding author. Endoscopic Skull Base Surgery Program, Otolaryngology Research, Rhinology and Sinus Surgery, Department of Otolaryngology–Head and Neck Surgery, Neurological Institute of New Jersey, Rutgers New Jersey Medical School, 90 Bergen Street, Suite 8100, Newark, NJ 07103.
E-mail address: jean.anderson.eloy@gmail.com

Otolaryngol Clin N Am 49 (2016) 951–964
http://dx.doi.org/10.1016/j.otc.2016.03.019
0030-6665/16/$ – see front matter © 2016 Elsevier Inc. All rights reserved.

Continued

- Newer techniques, such as balloon catheter dilation of the frontal sinus, offer a promising and less invasive alternative to more extensive frontal sinusotomies; however, practitioners should recognize their limitations based on individual experience with frontal sinus surgeries, and should not simply perform technically "easier" approaches in situations with complicated anatomy.
- If practitioners have limited comfort with these techniques in cases in which they are indicated, these patients would benefit from referral to surgeons with adequate experience in advanced frontal sinusotomy.

Abbreviations	
CSF	Cerebrospinal fluid
BCD	Balloon catheter dilation
ESS	Endoscopic sinus surgery
IGS	Image-guided surgery

INTRODUCTION

The increased utilization of endoscopic sinus surgery (ESS) over the past 30 years has triggered the development of novel approaches along with myriad accompanying technologies. Frontal sinus surgery in particular has undergone an evolution from being among the most extensive of paranasal sinus procedures to a predominantly outpatient, minimally invasive undertaking. Nonetheless, the intimate proximity of the frontal sinus to the skull base and orbit means frontal sinus surgery is still fraught with considerable potential morbidities, rendering a smaller margin for error relative to other sinonasal locations. Although recent advances in optical technologies and instrumentation have improved visualization and improved access, the frontal sinus outflow tract can still be easily disrupted. The rapid proliferation of new technologies over the past 10 years, including drug delivery and balloon catheter dilation (BCD) systems, further reinforces the importance of familiarity with anatomic considerations unique to the frontal sinuses. This review focuses on complications in frontal sinus surgery, both those specific to the frontal sinuses and those similar to the other sinuses, as well as strategies for avoiding deleterious sequelae. Rather than providing an exhaustive review of every possible complication, we focus on the most frequent and impactful complications in the context of common surgical techniques. Our hope is that this review serves as a useful resource for sinus surgeons at all levels, including the resident in training, rhinology fellow, general otolaryngologist, and experienced rhinologist.

PREOPERATIVE EVALUATION
Patient Selection and Counseling

As in all surgical procedures, appropriate patient selection is key for avoidance of harmful sequelae. Practitioners should ensure that patients undergoing any frontal sinus procedure have exhausted adequate medical management options. With few exceptions, surgical intervention should be considered only after unsuccessful or partially effective medical treatment has been undertaken.[1] Exceptions include but are not limited to obvious anatomic and structural features interfering with frontal sinus outflow tract, suspicion for neoplasm, frontal sinusitis with impending complications and consideration of other lesions, such as mucoceles, that may have local effects on surrounding critical structures.

Appropriate preoperative counseling is an important step for increasing patient understanding and comfort with surgical intervention. Engaging in a 2-way comprehensive discussion detailing risks, alternatives, and benefits not only improves patient satisfaction, but also facilitates postoperative adherence necessary for a successful outcome. Illustrative of this principle, complaints of inadequate informed consent are among the most consistently cited allegations in litigation related to rhinologic procedures.[2–8]

Preoperative Review of Imaging

In addition to exhibiting symptomatology and potentially exhausting medical management, there should be documentation of frontal sinusitis via either nasal endoscopy and/or imaging. For chronic disease, imaging is mandatory and can provide important information regarding individual anatomic variation that may impact surgical planning. In addition to evaluating the insertion of the uncinate process, as well as skull base anatomy, including Keros classification, there are several considerations specific to frontal sinus intervention (**Box 1**).[1,9–11] It is important to note the anatomy of the frontal sinus outflow tract, specifically identifying the presence of agger nasi cells, suprabullar cells, supraorbital ethmoid cells, and frontal cells (**Fig. 1**).[12] The presence of these cells, as well as other processes, such as osteoneogenesis, can impact the extent of frontal sinusotomy, and may also steer the surgeon away from less advanced approaches such as BCD.[13,14] Preoperative imaging also may be used to determine the necessity for image-guided surgery (IGS) during frontal sinus surgery.[15]

Hemostasis

In addition to general overall medical fitness for anesthesia, another factor for consideration is the likelihood of intraoperative hemorrhage. Excessive bleeding and consequently decreased visualization can significantly increase the probability of encountering the complications described later in this article. Hence, the preoperative evaluation should include comprehensive questioning regarding a personal and family history of bleeding diatheses. Further workup, including measurement of coagulation factors, should be undertaken if positive history of bleeding diathesis is elicited.

Optimal visualization is essential for success in ESS, particularly for frontal sinus procedures. Preoperative treatment with vasoconstrictive agents, both topical and infiltrative, is crucial for achieving this goal. Strategies for achieving hemostasis and locations for injection vary tremendously among institutions and practitioners.[16–19]

Box 1
Anatomic considerations on the preoperative imaging for endoscopic frontal sinus surgery

- Attachment of uncinate process
- Frontal sinus asymmetry
- Frontal sinus pneumatization
- Lamina papyracea dehiscence
- Location of extracranial anterior ethmoid artery
- Presence of nasoethmoid cells (agger nasi, suprabullar, supraorbital, frontal cells)
- Presence of osteoneogenesis

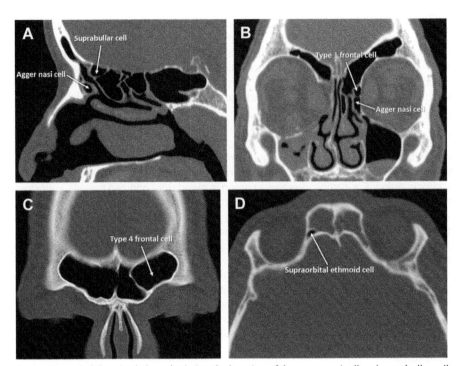

Fig. 1. CT scan in (A) sagittal plane depicting the location of the agger nasi cell and suprabullar cell. (B) CT scan in the coronal plane demonstrating a left type 1 frontal cell. (C) Coronal CT scan depicting a left type 4 frontal cell. (D) Axial CT scan demonstration of a right supraorbital ethmoid cell.

INTRAOPERATIVE TECHNIQUES AND RELEVANT ANATOMY

Due to the relative novelty of advanced techniques in frontal sinus surgery, there are few sizeable cohorts reporting the rates of specific complications. One single institution analysis retrospectively evaluating approximately 200 patients over a 20-year period noted permanent and "major" complications occurring in 2.7% of patients.[9,20] Importantly, the remarkable breadth in advances during this time period makes it unclear as to what extent this rate is associated with newer techniques and technologies. Complications discussed in this article are summarized in **Table 1**.

Endoscopic Endonasal Frontal Sinusotomy: Basic and Advanced Approaches and Potential Complications

Optimizing visualization through sound technique, such as ensuring appropriate hemostasis and holding an endoscope at the correct position, is paramount in preventing intraoperative disorientation that can complicate endoscopic frontal sinusotomy. Familiarity with the endoscopic frontal sinus anatomy is key in successfully undertaking this endeavor. To review briefly, going superior to the anterior border of a maxillary antrostomy, the frontal sinus can be identified at approximately 1 cm posterior to the anterosuperior attachment of the middle turbinate.[21,22] One can typically locate the frontal sinus outflow tract by aiming a frontal sinus probe superior and medially away from the medial orbital wall to find the point of entry.

As noted previously, preoperative review of the computed tomography (CT) scan and familiarity with the frontal sinus and surrounding anatomy unique to each

Table 1
Summary of selected complications of endoscopic frontal sinus surgery

Complication	Prevention	Management
CSF leak	Avoid removal of the middle turbinate posterior to the coronal plane of frontal sinus posterior table Consider use of IGS in revision cases, cases in which disease is abutting the skull base, cases where compromise of posterior frontal sinus table is suspected	• Observation if low-output leak is noted postoperatively • Stool softeners, activity restriction • Multilayer closure
Orbital injury decompression	Evaluate preoperative imaging for dehiscent lamina papyracea, location of uncinate process attachment, location of anterior ethmoid artery	• Elevate head of bed • Removal of nasal packing • Steroids, mannitol • Lateral canthotomy/cantholysis • Endoscopic MOW
Persistent disease/scarring	Mucosal preservation in frontal sinus outflow tract, can be facilitated by avoidance of power tools; removing nasoethmoid cells, recognizing presence of agger nasi cells, other accessory cells; ensuring position in the true frontal sinus ostium before deploying balloons; confirming location via transillumination	• Medical management • Balloon sinus dilation • Draf frontal sinusotomy
Vascular injury/bleeding	Using appropriate preoperative hemostasis Recognizing location of extracranial anterior ethmoid artery	See above
Mucocele	Adequate mucosal handling during ESS	Marsupialization

Abbreviations: CSF, cerebrospinal fluid; ESS, endoscopic sinus surgery; IGS, image guidance system; MOW, medial orbital wall.

individual patient is important for facilitating a safe and successful endoscopic frontal sinusotomy. Intraoperatively, familiarity with the presence of an agger nasi cell is paramount. When present, they must be opened, and a probe can subsequently be used to palpate the posterior wall of the frontal sinus. Furthermore, the superior aspects of both agger nasi cells and suprabullar cells can then be fractured and removed to facilitate visualization of the frontal sinus infundibulum.[22] Failure to recognize an agger nasi cell or suprabullar cell is a mistake that is not uncommon; with this failure, particularly with balloon dilation techniques, the frontal sinus outflow tract may become more obstructed.[21]

Once the bony fragments comprising the agger nasi cell, suprabullar cells, or other frontal cells are downfractured, upbiting forceps can be used to remove these fragments. Adequate mucosal preservation is important in preventing postoperative scarring and stenosis. Many practitioners avoid the use of power tools in this area to facilitate mucosal preservation.[23] This is also a key strategy in the avoidance of long-term sequelae, such as frontal sinus mucocele formation. Sound technique at this stage is among the most important steps in preventing long-term restenosis of the frontal sinus outflow tract. After the surgeon is confident that the frontal recess has been cleared of disease and occluding cells, transillumination is an important step in confirming appropriate dissection. If transillumination is witnessed in the medial canthal region, it is likely that a supraorbital ethmoid cell rather than the frontal sinus was opened, and further dissection is required to complete the frontal sinusotomy. An important caveat to this is how the degree of frontal sinus pneumatization affects transillumination; a patient with a poorly pneumatized frontal sinus (on the side trans-illumination is being attempted) might not have the light showing up in the typical frontal sinus location.

In summary, the keys to success in the basic endoscopic frontal sinusotomy include comprehensive preoperative review of the CT scan and taking steps to optimize intra-operative visualization and prevent disorientation. Furthermore, other important keys for preventing postoperative scarring and outflow pathway obstruction include confirming not only that the frontal sinus outflow tract is free of disease, but that ethmoid cells (including supraorbital and agger nasi cells) and other frontal cells are adequately addressed.

Endoscopic endonasal frontal sinus surgery now extends beyond those techniques described previously. In recent decades, the Draf techniques for endoscopic frontal sinus surgery have been described and have increased in popularity.[24,25] Accompanying these approaches, however, are the similar potential complications relating to the frontal sinus outflow tract. In addition to appropriate preoperative planning, familiarity with these techniques is paramount for success, and individuals with limited experience in extended frontal sinusotomy approaches may consider avoiding performing these procedures.

The different Draf approaches result in progressively wider frontal sinus outflow tract,[9] and are described briefly (**Fig. 2**). A Draf I frontal sinusotomy was essentially described previously, and removes suprabullar, agger nasi, and other ethmoid cells interfering with the frontal sinus outflow tract while preserving the sinonasal mucosa. Draf IIA refers to removal of cells extending into the actual frontal sinus, producing a route of drainage between the lamina papyracea and middle turbinate.[25] This latter technique is helpful for unresolved disease after a failed Draf I sinusotomy. The Draf IIB extended frontal sinusotomy expands this outflow farther medially to the nasal septum, and involves removal of the anterior portion of the middle turbinate. In addition to preventing fibrosis and scarring by adhering to the principles of mucosal preservation as described earlier, disruption of skull base and subsequent cerebrospinal fluid (CSF) rhinorrhea and other intracranial sequelae are additional risks with the Draf IIB procedure. For prevention, the surgeon should ensure that middle turbinate resection is limited to the portion anterior to the coronal plane of the frontal sinus posterior table.

The Draf III, or modified Lothrop procedure, is a further extension of the IIB technique, resulting in unified outflow pathway draining both frontal sinuses. In addition to performing a Draf IIB procedure bilaterally (creating outflow tract from lamina papyracea to nasal septum), the intersinus septum and the superior portion of the nasal septum are excised.[9,25–27] Similar precautions should be undertaken as in any other frontal sinus procedure, including awareness of the location of the skull base and the orbit. Variations in the Draf procedures have been described by Eloy and colleagues,[28–34] and require the same type of precautions to prevent complications. Frontal sinus surgery series with appreciable numbers of patients are sparse, meaning the true complication rates are not known and likely vary based on characteristics relating to patient selection and surgeon experience.

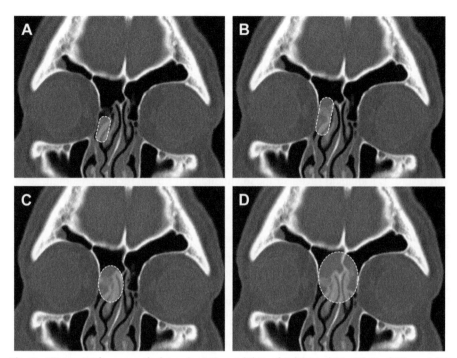

Fig. 2. CT scan in the coronal plane depicting a (*A*) Draf I, (*B*) Draf IIA, (*C*) Draf IIB, and (*D*) Draf III procedure. Teal areas depict the resected structures.

Frontal Sinus Balloon Catheter Dilation

There has been a dramatic increase in frontal sinus procedures concomitant with the advent and popularization of sinus balloon catheter technologies.[35,36] As the endoscopic management of advanced and severe frontal disease was previously considered "off limits" and fraught with hazard to practitioners without extensive experience, many have now become comfortable with the newer BCD approach due to its relative ease of use. The pros and cons of balloon catheter technology are beyond the scope of this article, but briefly, in addition to being less invasive than traditional frontal sinusotomies, these procedures can be performed in an outpatient in-office setting. The relative novelty of BCD of the sinuses means that the efficacy and cost-effectiveness of this strategy compared with traditional techniques is still unknown. A recent review by Batra[13] evaluating BCD overall noted that most available datasets lack controls and are retrospective, making comparison with ESS difficult. The review did reveal that there were data noting the ability of BCD, however, to result in frontal, sphenoid, and maxillary patency for up to 2 years. Nonetheless, there are limited studies with regard to longer-term patency rates, and there are several concerns regarding potential complications.

In terms of acute complications, BCD appears safe overall. In an analysis involving 628 patients undergoing in-office BCD of the sinuses, 5 (1.1%) of 468 patients with frontal sinus BCD experienced postprocedural bleeding, and only 1 (0.2%) sustained an orbital complication.[37] As these 6 patients with frontal sinus BCD who experienced complications also had dilation in other sinuses, these sequelae are unable to be attributed specifically to frontal sinus instrumentation; therefore, the real rates may have been lower.

Another potential complication associated with the use of BCD relates to dilation occurring in the wrong location. There is a significant potential for deploying the balloon in a manner that causes it to end up within an agger nasi or other frontoethmoidal cell, with dilation worsening frontal sinus outflow obstruction if performed improperly. This complication, once again, may be avoided by familiarity with the preoperative CT scan and the presence of these cells. Moreover, avoidance of the use of BCD in patients with certain anatomic variants may be prudent, as they may require a standard frontal sinusotomy. Heimgartner and colleagues[14] reported on their experience with BCD in 104 frontal sinuses.[13] Among the 12 cases with failure, CT imaging revealed these variations in frontal recess pneumatization, including agger nasi cells, frontoethmoidal cells, suprabullar cells, and the presence of osteoneogenesis.

External Approaches to Frontal Sinus Surgery

Advances in technology have significantly decreased the need for external frontal sinus surgery. There are several situations, however, in which external approaches are appropriate, whether as a primary strategy or an adjunct to endoscopic visualization. The main indications include disease involving the superior and/or lateral portions of the frontal sinus, anatomic difficulties, such as the presence of type 4 frontal cells, prior trauma, and osteomyelitis.[38–40]

Frontal sinus trephination is a relatively safe procedure, with complications relatively uncommon. The potential for a visible and unsightly scar is the most common and obvious disadvantage, and can be minimized by limiting the trephine used to 0.5 cm or less.[40,41] Paresthesias are also uncommon but possible due to potential supratrochlear nerve injury. Two other worrisome but easily avoidable complications of trephination are orbital and intracranial injury. Image guidance utilization may play a valuable role in avoidance of either of these injuries. For example, before performing the trephination, this technology can be used to identify the floor of the frontal sinus near its midline, where the posterior table is farthest away.[42] Other complications noted in large series detailing patients who underwent trephination revealed a small risk of facial cellulitis (2.1%–4.5%), as well the risk of uncommon sequelae of CSF leak and orbital complications.[39,43–45]

Although not commonly used anymore, the external frontoethmoidectomy is still being performed in some centers for select frontal, ethmoid, orbital, and skull base pathologies. Potential complications associated with this approach include lacrimal system dysfunction through stenosis of the nasolacrimal duct or direct injury to the lacrimal sac, hematomas through avulsion of the anterior ethmoid artery, optic nerve injury and visual loss if dissection is carried out too far posterior near the optic canal, and intracranial injury.

Frontal sinus osteoplastic flap obliteration has several additional complications in addition to those detailed for trephination. If a bicoronal approach is used, the surgeon should be familiar with the location of the frontal branch of the facial nerve, as failure to stay deep to the superficial temporal fascia may result in injury. Another complication specific to the osteoplastic flap is the potential for mucocele formation. The rate of mucocele formation is significant, and the importance of removing all grossly visible mucosa and further drilling to ensure removal of all remaining mucosa cannot be understated.[40] Mucoceles have been reported to occur decades after procedures, reinforcing the importance of prevention.

REVIEW OF SPECIFIC COMPLICATIONS
Cerebrospinal Fluid Leak

Intracranial injury represents a severe but fortunately uncommon occurrence in endoscopic frontal sinus surgery. Principles of prevention and management remain the same as in surgery of the other sinuses. By far the most common sequelae is CSF rhinorrhea, occurring in approximately 1 in 1000 patients undergoing any type of primary ESS.[46] As this is an exceedingly rare complication and there are few large series of patients undergoing frontal sinus ESS, whether the incidence of this complication is greater in frontal sinus cases is unclear. This injury can occur due to variations in skull base anatomy, leading to our recurring theme of familiarity with preoperative imaging. With regard to frontal sinus surgery specifically, disruption to the skull base can occur in procedures involving a Draf IIB frontal sinusotomy, as detailed previously. This typically occurs after resection of the anterior head of the middle turbinate posterior to the level of the frontal sinus posterior table. If a CSF leak is suspected intraoperatively, or if the clinical picture postoperatively is consistent with CSF rhinorrhea (as in patients with salty-tasting rhinorrhea, positional clear rhinorrhea, and so forth), there are several routes that may be pursued. Obvious or strongly suspected leak intraoperatively can be repaired with a variety of strategies, including a multilayer repair using a nasoseptal or turbinate-based flap, temporalis fascia, or allogeneic materials.[47–50] Postoperatively, patients with suspected CSF leaks can undergo β2-transferrin testing of their nasal drainage. Lower-output CSF leaks can be managed conservatively, whereas higher output and nonresolving leaks can be explored in the operating room, with consideration of preoperative intrathecal injection of fluorescein. The use of antibiotic prophylaxis for prevention of meningitis remains controversial.

Orbital Injury

Comprehensive preoperative planning and meticulous intraoperative technique are both important in preventing orbital complications in endoscopic frontal sinus surgery. Although the potential for orbital injury exists in ESS involving the other paranasal sinuses, the prevention and management of orbital complications takes on special importance on performance of frontal sinus surgery due to the intimate relationship of the orbit to the frontal sinus outflow tract and frontal sinus in general. The lamina papyracea represents the lateral border of the frontal sinus recess. Disruption of the medial orbital wall can result in several adverse sequelae variable in severity, including but not limited to asymptomatic herniation of orbital fat, orbital hematoma/hemorrhage, and extraocular muscle injury.[1,11]

Although there are few figures specific to frontal sinus surgery, orbital sequelae are relatively rare, with numerous analyses reporting rates far below 1%.[46,51–53] The CT scan should be inspected preoperatively for the attachment of the uncinate process; although not necessarily specific to frontal sinus surgery, this is important information to have in mind if an uncinectomy is planned.

Among the most severe complications, orbital hemorrhage can have a variable presentation, even encompassing blindness.[54] The appearance of this complication can significantly differ depending on whether the bleeding source is arterial or venous. In the case of the former, the anterior ethmoid artery is almost always the responsible vessel. One technique to avoid anterior ethmoid artery injury involves entering the frontal sinus by directing a probe away from the orbit *and* in an anterior direction away from the anterior ethmoid artery.[21,22] It is important to remember that the anterior ethmoid artery is typically 2 cm posterior to the middle turbinate's anterior attachment.[55] Anterior ethmoid artery injury can be associated with a coinjured superior oblique muscle, as they are in close proximity in a significant number of cases.[11,56] Key steps in the management of an arterial orbital hematoma include head elevation, removal of nasal packing if present, and emergent surgical management including lateral canthotomy with or without cantholysis, and endoscopic medial orbital wall decompression. In the case of a suspected venous bleed, with a slower presentation and less severe symptoms, conservative measures can be attempted with close observation and prompt ophthalmology consultation.

Preoperative imaging also should be inspected for defects in the lamina papyracea, as disruption of the medial orbital wall may result in serious consequences, including extraocular muscle damage. Disruption of the lamina papyracea may result in prolapse of orbital fat with exposure of the medial rectus muscle, which resultantly is the most commonly injured extraocular muscle. Extraocular muscle entrapment associated with lamina papyracea injury should be urgently managed with careful and meticulous debridement of fractured bony fragments. If complete medial rectus muscle transection is suspected, a variety of repair approaches may be taken by ophthalmologists. Even in cases that can be handled appropriately by otolaryngologists (ie, simple entrapment without muscle transection), ophthalmology involvement is paramount both from a medical and medicolegal perspective.[7,54,56,57]

Bleeding and Vascular Injury

The most common approaches for preventing complications related to bleeding are those detailed previously. Appropriate hemostasis intraoperatively is paramount in maintaining visualization during all endoscopic sinus cases, taking on even greater importance when working in the narrow area encompassing the frontal sinus outflow tract. Another important vascular consideration is familiarity with the location of the anterior ethmoid artery.

Mucocele Formation

The potential for mucocele formation after frontal sinusotomy was briefly discussed earlier in this article. Endoscopic management and marsupialization of mucoceles has become increasingly popular, although open approaches continue to be used. A recent meta-analysis noted comparable efficacy, and suggested that the persistence of a significant number of open cases may be related to a lack of expertise and equipment.[58] Nonetheless, Courson and colleagues[58] noted several discrete indications for open approaches, including unfavorable anatomy and lateral disease. Depending on expertise and comfort with frontal sinus procedures, advanced endoscopic approaches can be successful even in patients with those factors.[59,60] In lesions without complicating factors, BCD and drainage of a frontal sinus mucocele can be considered.[61,62] However, further studies are necessary to define the efficacy of this approach. Because of the proximity of the orbit and intracranial compartment to the frontal sinus, expanding mucocele of this region should be managed aggressively to prevent significant and sudden clinical impact.

SUMMARY

Novel technologies have facilitated the development of advanced surgical approaches to the frontal sinus in recent decades. Nonetheless, the intimate proximity of the frontal sinus to the skull base and orbit leaves a small margin for error. The frontal sinus outflow tract can be easily disrupted. Prevention of complications in frontal sinus surgery begins with appropriate preoperative assessment. With few exceptions, this includes ensuring that nonsurgical options have been exhausted, and that patients and physicians undergo dialogue discussing the potential for adverse events. For patients undergoing surgery, detailed preoperative evaluation of imaging for anatomic variants impacting the frontal sinus outflow tract is essential. Although newer techniques such as BCD offer a promising and less invasive alternative to the more extensive frontal sinusotomies, practitioners should recognize their limitations based on individual experience, and should not simply perform technically "easier" approaches in situations with complicated anatomy in which performance of more extensive techniques is warranted.

REFERENCES

1. Eloy JA, Svider PF, Setzen M. Clinical pearls in endoscopic sinus surgery: key steps in preventing and dealing with complications. Am J Otolaryngol 2014;35: 324–8.
2. Eloy JA, Svider PF, D'Aguillo CM, et al. Image-guidance in endoscopic sinus surgery: is it associated with decreased medicolegal liability? Int Forum Allergy Rhinol 2013;3:980–5.
3. Kovalerchik O, Mady LJ, Svider PF, et al. Physician accountability in iatrogenic cerebrospinal fluid leak litigation. Int Forum Allergy Rhinol 2013;3:722–5.
4. Re M, Magliulo G, Romeo R, et al. Risks and medico-legal aspects of endoscopic sinus surgery: a review. Eur Arch Otorhinolaryngol 2014;271:2103–17.
5. Stankiewicz JA, Hotaling J. Medicolegal issues in endoscopic sinus surgery and complications. Otolaryngol Clin North Am 2015;48:827–37.
6. Svider PF, Blake DM, Sahni KP, et al. Meningitis and legal liability: an otolaryngology perspective. Am J Otolaryngol 2014;35:198–203.
7. Svider PF, Kovalerchik O, Mauro AC, et al. Legal liability in iatrogenic orbital injury. Laryngoscope 2013;123:2099–103.
8. Svider PF, Mauro AC, Eloy JA, et al. Malodorous consequences: what comprises negligence in anosmia litigation? Int Forum Allergy Rhinol 2014;4:216–22.
9. Folbe AJ, Svider PF, Eloy JA. Advances in endoscopic frontal sinus surgery. Operat Tech Otolaryngol Head Neck Surg 2014;25:180–6.
10. Elwany S, Medanni A, Eid M, et al. Radiological observations on the olfactory fossa and ethmoid roof. J Laryngol Otol 2010;124:1251–6.
11. Svider PF, Baredes S, Eloy JA. Pitfalls in sinus surgery: an overview of complications. Otolaryngol Clin North Am 2015;48:725–37.
12. Wormald PJ. The agger nasi cell: the key to understanding the anatomy of the frontal recess. Otolaryngol Head Neck Surg 2003;129:497–507.
13. Batra PS. Evidence-based practice: balloon catheter dilation in rhinology. Otolaryngol Clin North Am 2012;45:993–1004.
14. Heimgartner S, Eckardt J, Simmen D, et al. Limitations of balloon sinuplasty in frontal sinus surgery. Eur Arch Otorhinolaryngol 2011;268:1463–7.
15. Ramakrishnan VR, Orlandi RR, Citardi MJ, et al. The use of image-guided surgery in endoscopic sinus surgery: an evidence-based review with recommendations. Int Forum Allergy Rhinol 2013;3:236–41.
16. Lee TJ, Huang CC, Chang PH, et al. Hemostasis during functional endoscopic sinus surgery: the effect of local infiltration with adrenaline. Otolaryngol Head Neck Surg 2009;140:209–14.
17. Moshaver A, Lin D, Pinto R, et al. The hemostatic and hemodynamic effects of epinephrine during endoscopic sinus surgery: a randomized clinical trial. Arch Otolaryngol Head Neck Surg 2009;135:1005–9.

18. Orlandi RR, Warrier S, Sato S, et al. Concentrated topical epinephrine is safe in endoscopic sinus surgery. Am J Rhinol Allergy 2010;24:140–2.

19. Eloy JA, Kovalerchik O, Bublik M, et al. Effect of greater palatine canal injection on estimated blood loss during endoscopic sinus surgery. Am J Otolaryngol 2014;35:1–4.

20. Hoskison E, Daniel M, Daudia A, et al. Complications of endoscopic frontal sinus surgery. Otolaryngol Head Neck Surg 2010;143(suppl 2):272.

21. Casiano RR. "Frontal sinusotomy" in endoscopic sinus surgery dissection manual. New York: Marcel Dekker, Inc; 2002.

22. Sargi ZB, Casiano RR. Surgical anatomy of the paranasal sinuses. In: Kountakis SE, Onerci M, editors. Rhinologic and sleep apnea surgical techniques. Heidelberg (Germany): Springer-Verlag; 2007. p. 17–26.

23. Javer AR, Alandejani T. Prevention and management of complications in frontal sinus surgery. Otolaryngol Clin North Am 2010;43:827–38.

24. Draf W, Weber R, Keerl R, et al. Current aspects of frontal sinus surgery. I: endonasal frontal sinus drainage in inflammatory diseases of the paranasal sinuses. HNO 1995;43:352–7 [in German].

25. Weber R, Draf W, Kratzsch B, et al. Modern concepts of frontal sinus surgery. Laryngoscope 2001;111:137–46.

26. Casiano RR, Livingston JA. Endoscopic Lothrop procedure: the University of Miami experience. Am J Rhinol 1998;12:335–9.

27. Gross WE, Gross CW, Becker D, et al. Modified transnasal endoscopic Lothrop procedure as an alternative to frontal sinus obliteration. Otolaryngol Head Neck Surg 1995;113:427–34.

28. Eloy JA, Friedel ME, Murray KP, et al. Modified hemi-Lothrop procedure for supraorbital frontal sinus access: a cadaveric feasibility study. Otolaryngol Head Neck Surg 2011;145:489–93.

29. Eloy JA, Kuperan AB, Friedel ME, et al. Modified hemi-Lothrop procedure for supraorbital frontal sinus access: a case series. Otolaryngol Head Neck Surg 2012; 147:167–9.

30. Liu JK, Mendelson ZS, Dubal PM, et al. The modified hemi-Lothrop procedure: a variation of the endoscopic endonasal approach for resection of a supraorbital psammomatoid ossifying fibroma. J Clin Neurosci 2014;21:2233–8.

31. Eloy JA, Friedel ME, Kuperan AB, et al. Modified mini-Lothrop/extended draf IIB procedure for contralateral frontal sinus disease: a cadaveric feasibility study. Otolaryngol Head Neck Surg 2012;146:165–8.

32. Eloy JA, Friedel ME, Kuperan AB, et al. Modified mini-Lothrop/extended draf IIB procedure for contralateral frontal sinus disease: a case series. Int Forum Allergy Rhinol 2012;2:321–4.

33. Eloy JA, Liu JK, Choudhry OJ, et al. Modified subtotal Lothrop procedure for extended frontal sinus and anterior skull base access: a cadaveric feasibility study with clinical correlates. J Neurol Surg B Skull Base 2013;74:130–5.

34. Eloy JA, Mady LJ, Kanumuri VV, et al. Modified subtotal-Lothrop procedure for extended frontal sinus and anterior skull-base access: a case series. Int Forum Allergy Rhinol 2014;4:517–22.

35. Psaltis AJ, Soler ZM, Nguyen SA, et al. Changing trends in sinus and septal surgery, 2007 to 2009. Int Forum Allergy Rhinol 2012;2:357–61.

36. Svider PF, Sekhsaria V, Cohen DS, et al. Geographic and temporal trends in frontal sinus surgery. Int Forum Allergy Rhinol 2015;5:46–54.

37. Sillers MJ, Lay KF, Holy CE. In-office balloon catheter dilation: analysis of 628 patients from an administrative claims database. Laryngoscope 2015;125:42–8.

38. Hahn S, Palmer JN, Purkey MT, et al. Indications for external frontal sinus procedures for inflammatory sinus disease. Am J Rhinol Allergy 2009;23:342–7.
39. Patel AB, Cain RB, Lal D. Contemporary applications of frontal sinus trephination: a systematic review of the literature. Laryngoscope 2015;125:2046–53.
40. Schneider JS, Day A, Clavena M, et al. Early practice: external sinus surgery and procedures and complications. Otolaryngol Clin North Am 2015;48:839–50.
41. Bent JP 3rd, Spears RA, Kuhn FA, et al. Combined endoscopic intranasal and external frontal sinusotomy. Am J Rhinol 1997;11:349–54.
42. Lee AS, Schaitkin BM, Gillman GS. Evaluating the safety of frontal sinus trephination. Laryngoscope 2010;120:639–42.
43. Batra PS, Citardi MJ, Lanza DC. Combined endoscopic trephination and endoscopic frontal sinusotomy for management of complex frontal sinus pathology. Am J Rhinol 2005;19:435–41.
44. Seiberling K, Jardeleza C, Wormald PJ. Minitrephination of the frontal sinus: indications and uses in today's era of sinus surgery. Am J Rhinol Allergy 2009;23: 229–31.
45. Walgama E, Ahn C, Batra PS. Surgical management of frontal sinus inverted papilloma: a systematic review. Laryngoscope 2012;122:1205–9.
46. Krings JG, Kallogjeri D, Wineland A, et al. Complications of primary and revision functional endoscopic sinus surgery for chronic rhinosinusitis. Laryngoscope 2014;124:838–45.
47. Eloy JA, Kuperan AB, Choudhry OJ, et al. Efficacy of the pedicled nasoseptal flap without cerebrospinal fluid (CSF) diversion for repair of skull base defects: incidence of postoperative CSF leaks. Int Forum Allergy Rhinol 2012;2:397–401.
48. Hoffmann TK, El Hindy N, Muller OM, et al. Vascularised local and free flaps in anterior skull base reconstruction. Eur Arch Otorhinolaryngol 2013;270:899–907.
49. Liu JK, Schmidt RF, Choudhry OJ, et al. Surgical nuances for nasoseptal flap reconstruction of cranial base defects with high-flow cerebrospinal fluid leaks after endoscopic skull base surgery. Neurosurg Focus 2012;32:E7.
50. Smith JE, Ducic Y, Adelson RT. Temporalis muscle flap for reconstruction of skull base defects. Head Neck 2010;32:199–203.
51. Bhatti MT. Neuro-ophthalmic complications of endoscopic sinus surgery. Curr Opin Ophthalmol 2007;18:450–8.
52. Bhatti MT, Stankiewicz JA. Ophthalmic complications of endoscopic sinus surgery. Surv Ophthalmol 2003;48:389–402.
53. Ramakrishnan VR, Kingdom TT, Nayak JV, et al. Nationwide incidence of major complications in endoscopic sinus surgery. Int Forum Allergy Rhinol 2012;2:34–9.
54. Stankiewicz JA, Chow JM. Two faces of orbital hematoma in intranasal (endoscopic) sinus surgery. Otolaryngol Head Neck Surg 1999;120:841–7.
55. Lee WC, Ming Ku PK, van Hasselt CA. New guidelines for endoscopic localization of the anterior ethmoidal artery: a cadaveric study. Laryngoscope 2000; 110:1173–8.
56. Han JK, Higgins TS. Management of orbital complications in endoscopic sinus surgery. Curr Opin Otolaryngol Head Neck Surg 2010;18:32–6.
57. Dutton JJ. Orbital complications of paranasal sinus surgery. Ophthal Plast Reconstr Surg 1986;2:119–27.
58. Courson AM, Stankiewicz JA, Lal D. Contemporary management of frontal sinus mucoceles: a meta-analysis. Laryngoscope 2014;124:378–86.
59. Friedel ME, Li S, Langer PD, et al. Modified hemi-Lothrop procedure for supraorbital ethmoid lesion access. Laryngoscope 2012;122:442–4.

60. Sama A, McClelland L, Constable J. Frontal sinus mucocoeles: new algorithm for surgical management. Rhinology 2014;52:267–75.
61. Barrow EM, DelGaudio JM. In-office drainage of sinus mucoceles: an alternative to operating-room drainage. Laryngoscope 2015;125:1043–7.
62. Eloy JA, Shukla PA, Choudhry OJ, et al. In-office balloon dilation and drainage of frontal sinus mucocele. Allergy Rhinol (Providence) 2013;4:e36–40.

Balloon Catheter Dilation of the Frontal Sinus Ostium

Michael J. Sillers, MD[a,b,]*, Kristopher F. Lay, MD[a]

KEYWORDS

- Balloon catheter dilation • Frontal sinus ostium • Medically refractory

KEY POINTS

- The decision to operate on the frontal sinus is based on persistent symptoms that have been refractory to appropriate medical therapy with associated radiographic evidence of disease by computed tomography.
- There is currently no evidence to support operating on radiographically negative frontal sinuses, regardless of the availability of technology or site of service options.
- There are many surgical procedures as well as a variety of different technologies available for the treatment of symptomatic, medically refractory frontal sinus disease.
- Balloon catheter dilation of the frontal sinus outflow tract allows for sinus ostial dilation with the option to spare tissue as a stand-alone procedure or as an adjunct to traditional endoscopic sinus surgery.
- Balloon catheter dilation can be performed safely in an office setting with outcomes comparable to those in traditional operating room settings.

INTRODUCTION

The surgical treatment of medically refractory frontal sinus disease offers a unique opportunity to significantly improve patients' quality of life.[1] The decision to operate on the frontal sinus outflow tract should not be made without great thought. This anatomic region can be quite complex, is normally narrow, and tends to scar easily when mucosa is not handled with care. Included in the thought process of recommending frontal sinus surgery should be an understanding of the underlying abnormality (inflammatory vs neoplastic), the unique anatomy of the frontal recess, the need for adequate exposure, the impact of the particular procedure on long-term postoperative follow-up, and the unique features of a wide array of surgical instrumentation

Disclosures: M.J. Sillers is a former member of Acclarent, Inc Scientific Advisory Board and has no financial disclosures. K.F. Lay has no disclosures.
[a] Alabama Nasal and Sinus Center, 7191 Cahaba Valley Road, Suite 301, Birmingham, AL 35242, USA; [b] Otolaryngology–Head and Neck Surgery, The University of Alabama-Birmingham, 2000, 6th Avenue South, Birmingham, AL, USA
* Corresponding author. Alabama Nasal and Sinus Center, 7191 Cahaba Valley Road, Suite 301, Birmingham, AL 35242.
E-mail address: mjsillers@gmail.com

available. Innovation and technology have significantly increased the specific surgical options for medically refractory disease in the frontal sinus. In general, balloon catheter dilation (BCD) has been shown to produce durable ostial patency. However, ostial patency alone may not be enough to assure an ideal outcome. Perhaps the most important factor in the choice of procedure and tools is a thorough understanding of the nature of the disease process. In stand-alone BCD procedures, there is no tissue removal. Therefore, if there is suspicion for or documentation of neoplastic disease, stand-alone BCD is contraindicated. Stand-alone BCD may also not be sufficient in patients with polyps or eosinophilic disease, where tissue removal is often necessary and where widening of the outflow tract by removing frontal recess cells facilitates local drug delivery. Finally, although there may be limited evidence that dilating a radiographically normal maxillary sinus improves symptoms,[2] there is currently no evidence for operating on a radiographically normal frontal sinus. Although there may be anecdotal reports of improved headaches, there is no evidence to support using BCD or any other instrumentation to operate on frontal sinuses without inflammatory disease.

The purpose of this article is to discuss the indications, relative contraindications, and techniques for using BCD of the frontal sinus outflow tract. It is important to state at the onset that the decision to intervene surgically is not instrument or site of service dependent. Before consideration for surgery, patients should have failed appropriate medical therapy, have persistent symptoms, and demonstrate abnormality on computed tomography (CT).

In general, BCD offers the unique opportunity to achieve durable sinus ostial and outflow tract dilation while sparing tissue in the process.[3-8] Specifically for the frontal sinus outflow tract, this technology allows for fracturing and lateral displacement of the medial and superior wall of obstructing frontal cells, medial displacement of an obstructing intersinus septal cell wall, and/or dilating soft tissue stenosis in previously operated patients (**Figs. 1** and **2**). Luong and colleagues[9] have reported on isolated BCD of the frontal sinus in the office setting. Using topical anesthesia, they found

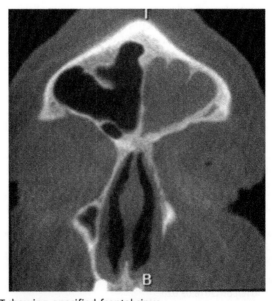

Fig. 1. Coronal CT showing opacified frontal sinus.

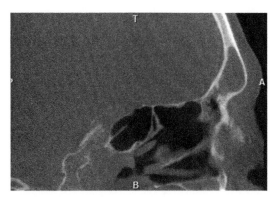

Fig. 2. Sagittal CT showing soft tissue obstruction of the frontal sinus infundibulum.

that durable patency was achieved in all 6 frontal sinuses dilated, with only one patient requiring a second dilation.

The largest study to date including in-office BCD of the frontal sinuses reported that 251 of 268 frontal sinuses were successfully dilated (93.7%) with 5 frontal sinuses requiring revision procedures (2%).[10]

Chan and colleagues[11] and Askar and colleagues[12] reported separately on 294 and 100 frontal sinuses operated using traditional functional endoscopic sinus surgery (FESS) techniques. Long-term patency was achieved in 88% and 90%, respectively. At first glance, it would appear the BCD achieves higher patency rates. However, patients undergoing BCD generally have a lower burden of disease than those undergoing traditional FESS procedures; this points to the importance of carefully selecting the appropriate procedure for the unique clinical situation.

Relative contraindications for BCD as a stand-alone procedure include cases where the underlying histology is in question, dense neo-osteogenesis of the frontal sinus outflow tract where sufficient displacement of bony walls is unlikely, and extensive polyposis. In these cases, traditional instrumentation should either be used to complement BCD technology or in its stead. Also, as stated previously, operating on frontal sinuses in the absence of demonstrable disease is not indicated regardless of the technology or site of service options.

An additional consideration for BCD is the ability to use this technology in the office setting. Office setting utilization has the obvious advantages of the elimination of the risks and recovery of general anesthesia and avoidance of cost associated with it and with the hospital outpatient department or ambulatory surgical facility. Proper patient selection is paramount. At minimum, patients should tolerate rigid diagnostic nasal endoscopy in the office setting before proceeding with in-office BCD.[13] In-office BCD has been shown to be safe and well tolerated with outcomes similar to those achieved in traditional venues.[10,14,15]

DEVICES

There are currently 3 manufacturers of US Food and Drug Administration–approved devices for BCD of the frontal, maxillary, and sphenoid sinuses. Acclarent, Inc (Menlo Park, CA, USA), Entellus (Plymouth, MN, USA), and Medtronic (Minneapolis, MN, USA) each have devices specifically designed for some of the unique features of frontal sinus outflow tract anatomy. Path Assist (**Fig. 3**) and Scout (**Fig. 4**) are designed to mimic a frontal seeker and are quite helpful in patients who have undergone prior surgery. Having the ability to change the trajectory of the tip of the wire is essential to

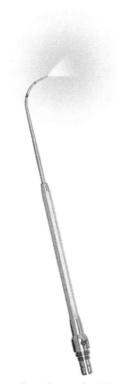

Fig. 3. Path assist. (*Courtesy of* Entellus, Plymouth, MN; with permission.)

proper ostial cannulation and subsequent balloon advancement and dilation of the frontal sinus outflow tract. Spin (**Fig. 5**) has the unique feature of a guide wire that the surgeon can literally "spin" and change the wire trajectory, which is quite helpful when multiple ostia are present in the frontal recess. Express (**Fig. 6**) has a malleable tip feature that can be very helpful in providing the proper angle for wire and balloon advancement and subsequent dilation. NuVent is a navigable device manufactured by Medtronic and is available for the frontal, maxillary, and sphenoid sinuses. The frontal

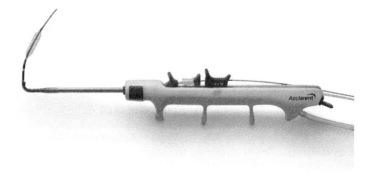

Fig. 4. Scout. (*Courtesy of* Acclarent, Irvine, CA; with permission.)

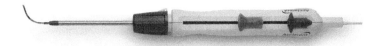

Fig. 5. Spin. (*Courtesy of* Acclarent, Irvine, CA; with permission.)

balloon (**Fig. 7**) is also similar to a frontal sinus seeker, and the tip is navigable with the Medtronic Fusion surgical navigation system.

TECHNIQUES

Techniques for successful balloon catheter advancement and frontal sinus outflow tract dilation vary depending on the patient's unique anatomy and/or history of prior surgery. In general, if BCD of multiple sinuses is planned, dilating the sphenoid sinus, frontal sinus, and finally the maxillary sinus is preferred in that order. The rationale for this is that operating on the anterior sinuses first may produce bleeding that makes visualizing and accessing the sphenoid sinus difficult. Because maxillary dilation includes medial displacement of the uncinate process, visualizing and accessing the frontal recess may become problematic if maxillary dilation is done before frontal dilation. BCD has been shown to be safe and tolerable in a traditional operating room setting with general anesthesia as well as in the office under topical anesthesia.

Successful access and dilation and patient satisfaction in the office setting are directly related to achieving adequate anesthesia and requires patience and communication on the part of the surgeon and patient alike. Combinations of 4% lidocaine or 2% tetracaine coupled with topical oxymetazoline or adrenalin on cotton pledgets have been described. Local infiltrative anesthesia may also be used. Staining 1:1000 topical adrenalin with methylene blue or fluorescein will help minimize the catastrophic risk of inadvertent injection of concentrated adrenalin. Specifically for the frontal sinus, placement of cotton pledgets both medial and lateral to the middle turbinate is helpful and allows for gentle medial displacement of the middle turbinate once anesthesia is achieved. Adequate anesthesia is often achieved when the patient reports dental numbness, which generally occurs 10 to 15 minutes following proper placement of the anesthetic.

Beginning with a 0° endoscope, the patient's nasal cavity is examined, and the middle turbinate is gently medialized with a Cottle or Freer elevator. The frontal recess is inspected with a 30° or 45° angled endoscope (**Fig. 8**). In the previously operated patient, a frontal sinus otium seeker or a seeker like balloon such as the Path Assist or Nuvent may be used to palpate a stenosed outflow tract or gently break through a soft tissue

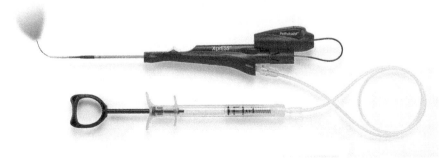

Fig. 6. Express. (*Courtesy of* Entellus, Plymouth, MN; with permission.)

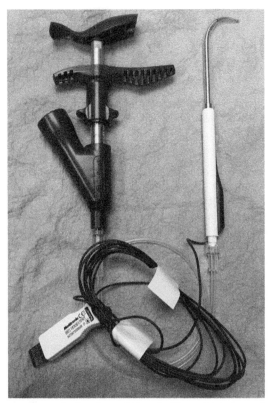

Fig. 7. Medtronic NuVent navigable frontal sinus balloon. (*Courtesy of* Medtronic, Minneapolis, MN; with permission.)

scar. Light assistance is helpful in transillumination of the frontal sinus once Path Assist or Scout is properly advanced. Transillumination is not always reliable. Transilluminating a supraorbital ethmoid air cell, Agger nasi cell, or a type III/IV frontal cell may incorrectly assure proper frontal sinus access. For this reason, using surgical navigation with NuVent

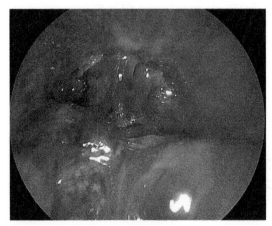

Fig. 8. Endoscopic view of scarred frontal sinus ostium.

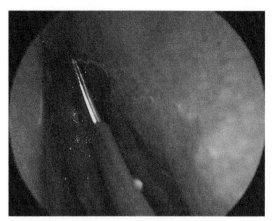

Fig. 9. Guidewire advanced into the frontal recess.

may be preferable in situations where the patient's unique anatomy may be complex. At this point, the guidewire is advanced into the frontal sinus (**Fig. 9**). Once proper placement of the device is confirmed, an appropriate diameter and length balloon is advanced (**Fig. 10**) and dilated to 10 to 12 atm of pressure (**Fig. 11**). In the awake patient (in the operating room or office), balloon dilation is the moment that intense pain may be reported. Communicating this in advance is essential. Balloon inflation generally lasts a few seconds, and patients have reported this as a tolerable event in the overwhelming majority of instances. In patients with simple narrowing or soft tissue stenosis, a single dilation may be sufficient. However, in cases with a more lengthy obstruction, such as a type III frontal cell medial wall, 2 or more dilations may be necessary to adequately reestablish a patent frontal sinus outflow tract (**Fig. 12**).

Following dilation, irrigation can be performed through a variety of catheters that may be advanced into the sinus, and secretions may be collected for appropriate studies. At this point, the adequacy of the dilation is assessed, and the sinusotomy may be enlarged with traditional instrumentation (**Fig. 13**). On completion of the procedure, the patient is observed for acute complications and discharged. Packing is

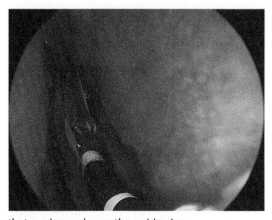

Fig. 10. Balloon catheter advanced over the guidewire.

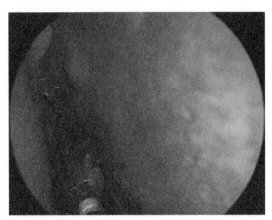

Fig. 11. Proximal balloon dilation.

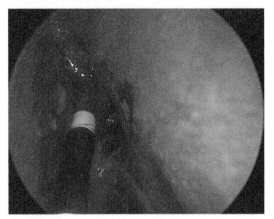

Fig. 12. Distal balloon dilation.

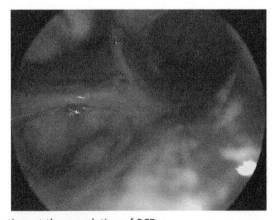

Fig. 13. Frontal ostium at the completion of BCD.

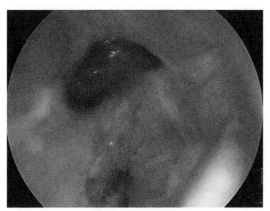

Fig. 14. Patent frontal sinus outflow tract 3 months after procedure.

rarely required. Patients should undergo endoscopic follow-up as with traditional FESS, and the durability of the ostial dilation can be assessed (**Fig. 14**).

SUMMARY

Balloon catheter dilatation represents an evolving technology that complements existing surgical instrumentation for the treatment of medically refractory chronic rhinosinusitis. As with any surgical procedure, appropriate selection of technique, instrumentation, and even site of service is guided by the disease process, underlying anatomy, and patient tolerability. Rhinologic surgeons should carefully appraise new technology and be willing to evolve thought processes in the treatment of a benign disease process that may have a significant impact on patients' quality of life.

REFERENCES

1. Naidoo Y, Bassiouni A, Keen M, et al. Risk factors for outcomes for primary, revision, and modified Lothrop (Draf III) frontal sinus surgery. Int Forum Allergy Rhinol 2013;3:412–7.
2. Bikazi A, Taulu R, Numminen J, et al. Quality of life after endoscopic sinus surgery or balloon sinuplasty: a randomized clinical study. Rhinology 2014;52(4):300–5.
3. Bolger W, Brown C, Church C, et al. Safety and outcomes of balloon catheter sinusotomy: a multi-center 24 week analysis in 115 patients. Otolaryngol Head Neck Surg 2007;137:10–20.
4. Levine H, Sertich A II, Hoisington D, et al. A multicenter registry of balloon catheter sinusotomy outcomes for 1036 patients. Ann Otol Rhinol Laryngol 2008;117: 263–70.
5. Weiss R, Church C, Kuhn F, et al. Long-term outcome analysis of balloon catheter sinusotomy: two-year follow-up. Otolaryngol Head Neck Surg 2008;139:S38–46.
6. Stankiewicz J, Truitt T, Atkins J. One-year results: transantral balloon dilation of the ethmoid infundibulum. Ear Nose Throat 2010;89:72–7.
7. Stankiewicz J, Truitt T, Winegar B, et al. Two-year results: antral dilation of the ethmoid infundibulum. Int Forum Allergy Rhinol 2012;2(3):199–206.
8. Kutluhan A, Bozdemir K, Cetin H, et al. Endoscopic balloon dilation sinuplasty including ethmoidal air cells in chronic rhinosinusitis. Ann Otol Rhinol Laryngol 2009;118(12):881–6.

9. Luong A, Batra P, Fakhri S, et al. Balloon catheter dilation for frontal sinus ostium stenosis in the office setting. Am J Rhinol 2008;22(6):621–4.

10. Karanfilov B, Silvers S, Pasha R, et al. Office-based balloon sinus dilation: a prospective multi-center study of 203 patients. Int Forum Allergy Rhinol 2013;3: 404–11.

11. Chan Y, Melroy C, Kuhn C, et al. Long-term frontal sinus patency after endoscopic frontal sinusotomy. Laryngoscope 2009;119(6):1229–32.

12. Askar M, Gamea A, Tomoum M, et al. Endoscopic management of chronic frontal rhinosinusitis: prospective quality of life analysis. Ann Otol Rhinol Laryngol 2015; 124(8):638–48.

13. Prickett K, Wise S, DelGaudio J. Cost analysis of office-based and operating room procedures in rhinology. Int Forum Allergy Rhinol 2012;2:207–11.

14. Albritton F, Casiano R, Sillers M. Feasability of in-office endoscopic sinus surgery with balloon sinus dilation. Am J Rhinol Allergy 2012;26(3):243–8.

15. Cutler J, Truitt T, Atkins J, et al. First clinic experience: patient selection and outcomes for ostial dilation for chronic rhinosinusitis. Int Forum Allergy Rhinol 2011; 1(6):460–5.

Utility of Image-Guidance in Frontal Sinus Surgery

 CrossMark

Gretchen M. Oakley, MD[a],*, Henry P. Barham, MD[c], Richard J. Harvey, MD, PhD[a,b,1]

KEYWORDS

- Frontal sinus • Frontal • Sinusitis • Rhinosinusitis • Image guidance • Navigation

KEY POINTS

- Image guidance is a surgical tool that is widely accepted by endoscopic surgeons and used in most frontal sinus surgeries.
- The use of image guidance can help identify critical structures and distorted anatomic landmarks, increasing the surgeon's confidence and ability to perform a more complete dissection.
- Image-guided placement of limited external frontal sinusotomy allows access to and management of frontal sinus disease that is beyond the endoscopic reach while avoiding the need for an osteoplastic flap.

BACKGROUND ON IMAGE GUIDANCE IN ENDOSCOPIC SINUS SURGERY

The use of image-guided surgery (IGS) in endoscopic sinus surgery (ESS) has expanded during the last 2 decades. A 2010 survey of American Rhinologic Society members[1] suggests that more surgeons have access to IGS and are using this technology in a greater percentage of cases compared with a similar survey conducted in 2005.[2] With respect to frontal sinus procedures, 71% of respondents thought there was a relative or absolute indication for its use in primary frontal sinus exploration, 96% in revision frontal sinus exploration, and 98% in modified Lothrop

Disclosure Statement: R.J. Harvey has served on an advisory board for Schering Plough and GlaxoSmithKline; has acted as a consultant for Medtronic, Olympus, and Stallergenes; has served on the speakers bureau for Merck Sharp Dohme and Arthrocare; and has received grant support from NeilMed Pharmaceuticals. G.M. Oakley and H.P. Barham has no conflicts of interest to declare pertaining to this article.
^a Rhinology and Skull Base Research Group, Applied Medical Research Centre, University of New South Wales, 405 Liverpool St, Sydney, NSW 2011, Australia; ^b Faculty of Medicine and Health Sciences, Macquarie University, Building F10A, Ground Floor, 2 Technology Pl., Sydney, NSW 2109, Australia; ^c Department of Otolaryngology Head and Neck Surgery, Louisiana State University, 433 Bolivar St, New Orleans, LA 70112, USA
¹ Present address: Ground Floor, 67 Burton Street, Darlinghurst, New South Wales 2010, Australia.
* Corresponding author. Ground Floor, 67 Burton Street, Darlinghurst, New South Wales 2010, Australia.
E-mail address: gmoakley@gmail.com

Otolaryngol Clin N Am 49 (2016) 975–988
http://dx.doi.org/10.1016/j.otc.2016.03.021
oto.theclinics.com

procedures.[1] Although it is well known that IGS is not a substitute for sound anatomic knowledge and clinical decision-making,[3] it may help minimize the risk of injury by verifying the location of vital structures surrounding the paranasal sinuses and assist in a more complete clearance of disease. Logically, this would translate into fewer surgical complications and improved patient outcomes, the former of which was a conclusion of a recent meta-analysis of surgical cohorts with and without IGS in sinus surgery.[4]

Complication rates for ESS have been reported to range from 0.36% to 3.1%.[5–7] Although all aspects of ESS can present challenges, surgery of the frontal sinus is the most technically demanding. The complex and varied anatomy, acute nasofrontal angle, and proximity to critical structures, such as the olfactory fossa, skull base, vascular structures (anterior ethmoid artery), and orbit contribute to the technical difficulty of frontal recess surgery. In addition, distorted anatomy from chronically inflamed mucosa and absent anatomic landmarks from prior surgery only add to the potential risk. However, IGS has uses well beyond simply avoiding complications. It can facilitate identifying the appropriate location for an external frontal trephine (or minitrephine), mapping an osteoplastic flap, or defining the extent of nasofrontal beak exposure before Draf III sinusotomy. Some procedures, such as an image-guided external biopsy of lateral frontal sinus disease, depend entirely on the IGS technology.

Image-guidance systems typically used in ESS can be either optically based or electromagnetic-based, and consist of a computer workstation, tracking system, and specially designed navigation instruments (**Fig. 1**). The patient's image-guidance compatible computed tomography (CT) scan, usually an axial noncontrast CT with 1 mm or thinner cuts, is loaded into the system either by CD-ROM or over a broadband network preoperatively. Once the image guidance is registered to the patient, intraoperative localization of a given navigation instrument is displayed in real time on the patient's preoperative CT in axial,

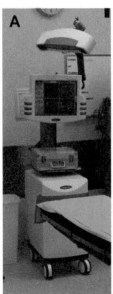
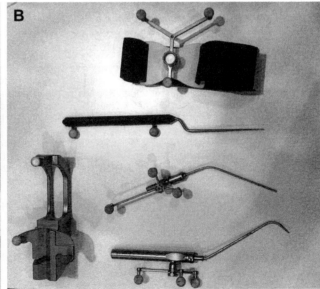

Fig. 1. Standard image guidance system used in ESS (*A*) with associated instrumentation (*B*).

coronal, and sagittal planes (**Fig. 2**). Image-guidance accuracy has been shown to be within 2 mm[8] and a variety of frontal sinus navigation instruments have been developed to make it well suited for this type of surgery. Although excellent for general localization or reorienting the surgeon, they are not accurate enough to help with submillimeter decision-making around critical skull base anatomy.

UTILITY OF IMAGE GUIDANCE IN ENDOSCOPIC SINUS SURGERY

Several studies directed at IGS use in ESS have been performed to analyze its associated complication rate, revision rate, patient quality of life outcomes, cost, and medicolegal role.[4,6,8–16]

Complications

In an evidence-based review with recommendations (EBRR) by Ramakrishnan and colleagues,[13] 6 studies reported complication rates in IGS compared with non-IGS

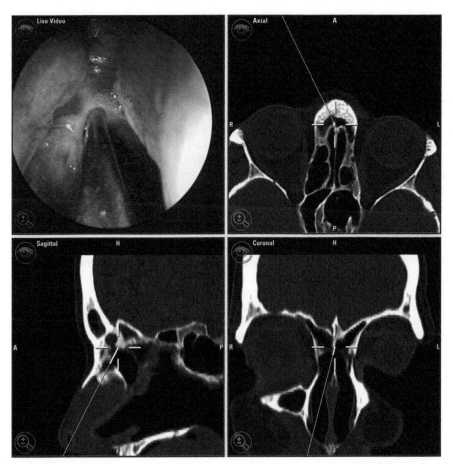

Fig. 2. Standard image guidance real-time view. The location of the tip of the probe is shown on the patient's preoperative CT scan in all 3 planes.

groups. Four of the 6 studies showed no statistically significant difference in compli-cation rates with IGS,[11,15–17] whereas 2 studies did show a significant difference in major complications with IGS use. One of these studies showed fewer major compli-cations with IGS use (intracranial injury, orbital injury, major hemorrhage, and aborted procedure) but no difference in minor complications (not specifically defined),[10] whereas the other actually showed an increased rate of orbital injuries with the use of IGS but no other significant differences.[6] There was determined to be a preponder-ance of benefit versus harm based on C-level quality of evidence, making the use of IGS for the reduction of complications an option. In a meta-analysis of 13 relevant studies, including 5 of the 6 studies in the previously mentioned EBRR, Dalgorf and colleagues[4] reported that the rate of major complications and total complications did favor the use of IGS with statistical significance when the data was pooled.

Revision Rate

In a retrospective review of 120 subjects who underwent ESS with use of IGS, 16.5% of subjects went on to require revision surgery, although there was no comparison group in this study.[15] Fried and colleagues[10] retrospectively reviewed 160 subjects and did report a significantly higher need for revision surgery in the non-IGS patient group than in the IGS group. However, a similarly designed study with 203 subjects had contradicting findings.[11] More recently, 2 separate meta-analyses found no signif-icant difference in subsequent revision rates with or without the initial use of IGS.[4,14]

Quality of Life Outcomes

Three studies compared subject quality of life outcomes after ESS with or without the use of IGS. One retrospective chart review found no difference in Sino-Nasal Outcome Test (SNOT)-20 scores at least 6 months after surgery.[15] Two prospective, non-randomized studies found conflicting results, 1 with improved Rhinosinusitis Outcome Measure (RSOM)-31 scores 6 months after IGS and the other with no difference in vi-sual analog scale (VAS) scores 12 months after IGS.[12,16] Although these studies show varied results individually, when their data were pooled by Dalgorf and colleagues[4] there was no evidence of a significant difference in quality of life outcomes whether or not IGS was used.

Cost and Medicolegal Concerns

The cost of IGS is an accumulation of the navigation system, disposable supplies or equipment costs, and any added operative time. One study reported that in otherwise similar subject groups, IGS was 6.7% more expensive than non-IGS.[11] They noted, however, that significant intangible benefits of this surgical adjunct may justify its use despite the increased cost but be too difficult to illustrate.

With respect to medicolegal situations, whether or not IGS was used did not play a role in ESS litigation initiation or outcomes from 2004 to 2013.[9] Case-specific factors and expert opinion from the operating surgeon should determine whether or not the cost and extra setup time is justified, instead of a habitual practice of defensive medicine.

The literature illustrating advantages or disadvantages of IGS is very limited. For example, to show a statistical difference in complication rate with IGS, power analyses have indicated that thousands of subjects would need to be enrolled in a prospective study.[16,18] That image guidance is currently widely accepted as being indicated in certain scenarios based on expert opinion makes future randomized studies (in which some subjects will be randomized away from IGS use even if the surgeon feels it is necessary) ethically impossible.[19] The American Academy of Otolaryngology–Head and Neck Surgery endorses the use of IGS during ESS in select cases guided by expert opinion, surgeon preference, and patient-specific factors. These indications are at the discretion of the surgeon and include revision surgery, distorted anatomy, extensive sinonasal polyposis, frontal or posterior sinus disease, disease-abutting vital structures, skull base defects, and neoplasms.[20]

ENDOSCOPIC USES OF IMAGE GUIDANCE
Maximizing the Frontal Sinusotomy

The frontal sinus and its outflow tract are known for variable anatomy, surrounding vital structures, and a narrow ostium predisposed to scarring and obstruction following surgical manipulation. The frontal recess is bordered medially by the middle turbinate, laterally by the lamina papyracea, anteriorly by the agger nasi cell, and posteriorly by the superior aspect of the ethmoid bulla along with the anterior ethmoid artery. In addition to the agger nasi cell anteriorly, there can be 1 or numerous frontal cells that sit above the agger nasi and pneumatize into the frontal recess, into the frontal sinus, or be isolated within the frontal sinus (**Fig. 3**A). Posteriorly and laterally to the frontal recess, patients can have frontal bullar cells or supraorbital cells that similarly encroach on the outflow space (**Fig. 3**B).

Frontal cells, supraorbital cells, and agger nasi cells can all be mistaken for the frontal recess.[21] Chiu and Vaughan[22] studied 67 subjects who were undergoing revision frontal sinus surgery to determine what led to their initial surgical failure and found that 79% had residual agger nasi and/or ethmoid bulla remnants; 49% had scarring of the frontal recess, often along with obstructing ethmoid cells or uncinate process (39%); 36% had lateralized middle turbinate remnants with scarring of the frontal recess; and 12% had unopened supraorbital ethmoid or frontal recess cells. In addition to careful preoperative planning with review of the patient's CT imaging, intraoperative image guidance can assist the surgeon in performing a more complete dissection, particularly in the setting of confusing frontal and supraorbital ethmoid cells.

IGS can help optimize the chances for success by assisting the surgeon in safely maximizing the final frontal recess dimensions. A completed Draf IIa frontal sinusotomy should be bound only by a clean lamina papyracea with no residual partitions, nasal beak, middle turbinate attachment, and the posterior table of the frontal sinus should be relatively continuous with the ethmoid roof and cribriform plate (**Fig. 4**). A

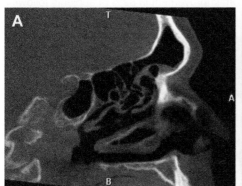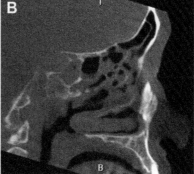

Fig. 3. (*A*) Sagittal view of a frontal recess that is narrowed anteriorly by the presence of a type III frontal cell, which sits atop the agger nasi and pneumatizes into the frontal sinus. (*B*) This frontal recess is narrowed posteriorly by a large frontal bullar cell, which is a pneumatized bulla lamella that extends into the frontal sinus.

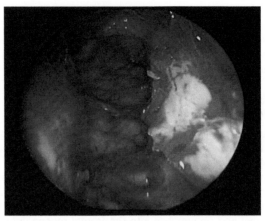

Fig. 4. Intraoperative view of a completed Draf IIa. The limits of dissection are shown, including lamina papyracea, nasal beak, middle turbinate attachment, and that the posterior table of the frontal sinus should be relatively continuous with the ethmoid roof and cribriform plate.

Draf IIb will be similar but with the medial border being septum rather than middle turbinate attachment. A Draf III (modified Lothrop) should have exposed nasal beak periosteum anteriorly, clean lamina papyracea bilaterally, and first olfactory neuron posteriorly (see later discussion). Critical structures such as the anterior ethmoid artery, skull base, and orbit can be verified intraoperatively during these dissections. This is particularly helpful in cases of dehiscent or low-hanging anterior ethmoid artery, asymmetric skull base, or dehiscent lamina papyracea (**Figs. 5** and **6**).

Modified Lothrop Procedure

The modified endoscopic Lothrop procedure is an established technique for managing recalcitrant inflammatory frontal sinus disease by reinstating drainage through a common pathway and providing much needed access for topical therapies. This procedure is also used for treating mucoceles, cerebrospinal fluid (CSF) leaks, and frontal or anterior skull base tumors. A systematic review with meta-analysis reported a success rate of 86% and significant symptom improvement in 82% of subjects following

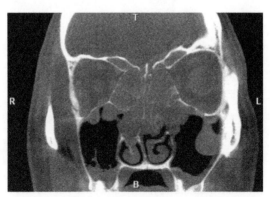

Fig. 5. Coronal CT scan showing low anterior ethmoid arteries. These are at risk of injury during frontal recess dissection if the surgeon is not aware of their location.

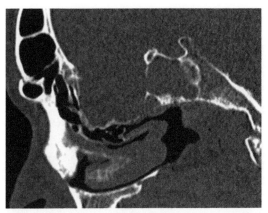

Fig. 6. Sagittal CT scan showing an asymmetric skull base. The asymmetry is secondary to a significant bony dehiscence with associated encephalocele.

modified Lothrop.[23] Since Professor Draf's first description of his approach to the common frontal sinusotomy, the landmarks of a frontal drillout remain unchanged.[24] However, endoscopically, the approach varies among surgeons and institutions. Image guidance is used in 80% of modified Lothrop procedures[23] to identify critical landmarks and distorted anatomy, particularly given that this patient population often has had multiple prior surgeries and ongoing sinonasal mucosal inflammation. Image guidance can be used in this setting to easily mark the site of the septal window (**Figs. 7** and **8**). The outside-in approach to the modified Lothrop uses fixed landmarks that are not easily distorted by disease, therefore maintaining easy surgical orientation.[25] The first olfactory neuron is a critical landmark to avoid the skull base and preserve olfactory bearing mucosa.[26] Early identification of the periosteum keeps the surgical field wide and ensures surgeon confidence in the bony removal. This technique leads to a safe and efficient opening of a wide Lothrop cavity (**Fig. 9**).

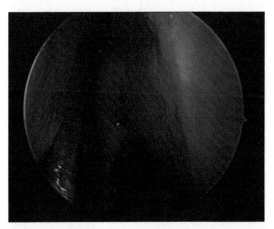

Fig. 7. Intraoperative view of image guidance used for help marking the septal window in an outside-in modified Lothrop procedure.

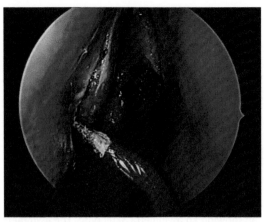

Fig. 8. Making the septal window as an initial step in the modified Lothrop procedure. The first olfactory neuron marks the posterior limit.

EXTERNAL USES OF IMAGE GUIDANCE
Limited or Directed External Sinusotomy

The increasing use of endoscopic approaches for paranasal sinus and skull base diseases has made the need for external approaches less and less common. However, there are limitations to what can be accessed endoscopically, so external approaches to frontal sinus disease still play an important role in management of certain disease processes. Perhaps the most common scenario is in the case of superior or lateral frontal sinus lesions, frequently mucoceles. Traditionally, these lesions would require an osteoplastic flap for surgical clearance. Directed external sinusotomy, or frontal trephination, is a more minimally invasive approach that can provide a portal for endoscopes and instruments to access isolated or superolateral lesions that otherwise do not require the wide access of an osteoplastic flap but cannot be reached from below.

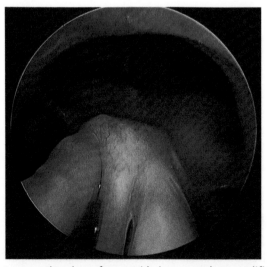

Fig. 9. The final intraoperative view after outside-in approach to modified Lothrop.

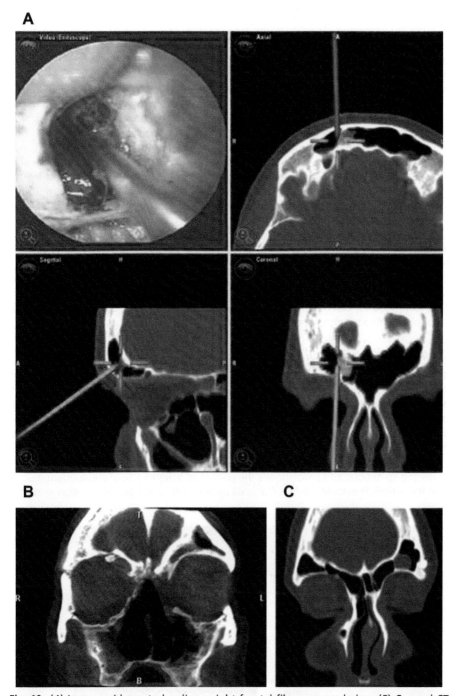

Fig. 10. (A) Image guidance to localize a right frontal fibro-osseous lesion. (B) Coronal CT scan of a lateral right frontal sinus mucocele. (C) Coronal CT scan showing an opacified type 4 frontal cell. All of these lesions can be accessed via directed external frontal sinusotomy.

Although surface anatomy can be used for a traditional external sinusotomy approach through the inferomedial portion of the anterior table of the frontal sinus, the use of image guidance helps mark the site with increased accuracy and can offer trajectory planning. Some examples of disease for which image-guided external frontal sinusotomy has been effective include fibro-osseous lesions, lateral mucoceles, type III or IV frontal cells (**Fig. 10**), and frontal recess stenosis or ossification.[27]

An added benefit of using image guidance is that it allows adjustment of the external sinusotomy site as needed to precisely target the frontal disease. Incisions can be hidden in the lateral brow or a forehead crease to keep cosmesis optimized, while keeping the safety margin high and still avoiding the added morbidity of the traditional osteoplastic flap (**Fig. 11**). In addition to allowing access to isolated disease beyond endoscopic reach or functioning as a portal for a combined above-and-below approach, a limited external frontal sinusotomy can also provide a direct route for an intersinus septectomy or even a frontal sinus obliteration if the sinuses are small enough.

Intersinus septectomy via limited external frontal sinusotomy has been described as a method to address unilateral frontal sinus disease when endoscopic techniques are not an option.[28,29] Frontal sinus drainage is reinstated by diverting it to the contralateral outflow tract (**Fig. 12**). Another use of IGS is to localize a posterior table fracture with associated CSF leak and position an external frontal sinusotomy for the repair. This technique for CSF leak repair can obviate standard frontal sinus obliteration via osteoplastic flap or intracranial approach.[30,31]

Defining the Osteoplastic Flap

If an osteoplastic flap is necessary, image guidance can precisely mark the edges of the sinus for the bony cuts. Although osteoplastic flap with frontal sinus obliteration has a high success rate at 93%,[32] there is a high risk of complications from the frontal bony cuts, such as dural exposure, dural injury with CSF leak, and orbital fat exposure.[33] The precision with which the sinus margins are identified is important because overestimating the margins leads to the previously mentioned complications. Alternatively, underestimating and leaving a bony lip makes complete obliteration of mucosa under the lip difficult and predisposes the patient to a higher risk of subsequent mucocele formation. Previously, 6-foot Caldwell radiography and transillumination were the

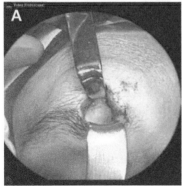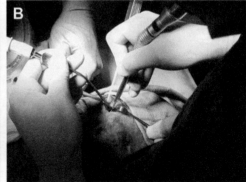

Fig. 11. (*A*) Intraoperative view of a directed external frontal sinusotomy incision positioned in the brow for optimal access and postoperative cosmetic results. (*B*) Drilling the external frontal sinusotomy.

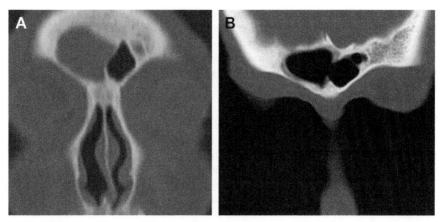

Fig. 12. (*A*) Preoperative and (*B*) 6 month postoperative coronal CT scans following intersinus septectomy to reinstate frontal sinus drainage through the contralateral outflow tract.

methods used to plan osteoplastic flap cuts. In the former, a radiograph is taken at a distance of 6 feet from the beam emitter at a 15° to 20° angle from the Frankfort plan, cut out of the film, sterilized, and placed on the patient's forehead and used to trace the frontal sinus.[34,35] In the latter, the frontal sinus margin is determined to be at the

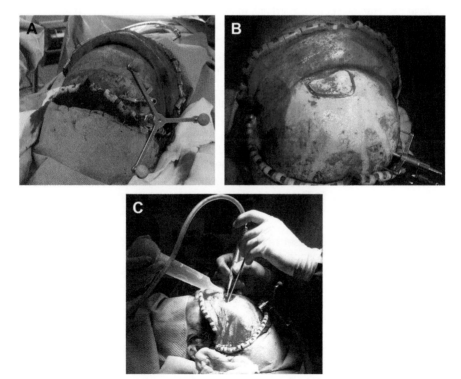

Fig. 13. A bicoronal incision is made for the osteoplastic flap approach (*A*). Image guidance is secured to the skull and used to identify the frontal sinus margins. The osteoplastic flap is then drilled (*B*), and the frontal sinus disease is addressed and the sinus is obliterated (*C*).

interface between light and dark areas of the frontal bone when shining a light externally or from the sinuses below.[34,36] Carrau and colleagues[37] were the first to describe frontal sinus mapping using image guidance in 1994, and studies comparing the efficacy of image guidance for this purpose with other methods, such as 6-foot Caldwell radiography and transillumination, have shown image guidance to be the most accurate and quickest[34,38,39] (Fig. 13).

SUMMARY

Image guidance is a surgical tool that helps verify vital structures and manage disorienting surgical conditions. Although it does not replace sound knowledge of anatomy, critical decision making, or technical expertise, it can improve surgeon confidence in performing safer surgery and more completely clearing disease. It has a variety of applications in endoscopic and external approach sinus surgery, and has contributed to the expanding role of endoscopic surgical approaches for paranasal sinus inflammatory and neoplastic disease.

REFERENCES

1. Justice JM, Orlandi RR. An update on attitudes and use of image-guided surgery. Int Forum Allergy Rhinol 2012;2(2):155–9.
2. Orlandi RR, Petersen E. Image guidance: a survey of attitudes and use. Am J Rhinol 2006;20(4):406–11.
3. Wise SK, Harvey RJ, Goddard JC, et al. Combined image guidance and intraoperative computed tomography in facilitating endoscopic orientation within and around the paranasal sinuses. Am J Rhinol 2008;22(6):635–41.
4. Dalgorf DM, Sacks R, Wormald PJ, et al. Image-guided surgery influences perioperative morbidity from endoscopic sinus surgery: a systematic review and meta-analysis. Otolaryngol Head Neck Surg 2013;149(1):17–29.
5. Krings JG, Kallogjeri D, Wineland A, et al. Complications of primary and revision functional endoscopic sinus surgery for chronic rhinosinusitis. Laryngoscope 2014;124(4):838–45.
6. Ramakrishnan VR, Kingdom TT, Nayak JV, et al. Nationwide incidence of major complications in endoscopic sinus surgery. Int Forum Allergy Rhinol 2012;2(1): 34–9.
7. Stankiewicz JA, Lal D, Connor M, et al. Complications in endoscopic sinus surgery for chronic rhinosinusitis: a 25-year experience. Laryngoscope 2011; 121(12):2684–701.
8. Metson R, Gliklich RE, Cosenza M. A comparison of image guidance systems for sinus surgery. Laryngoscope 1998;108(8 Pt 1):1164–70.
9. Eloy JA, Svider PF, D'Aguillo CM, et al. Image-guidance in endoscopic sinus surgery: is it associated with decreased medicolegal liability? Int Forum Allergy Rhinol 2013;3(12):980–5.
10. Fried MP, Moharir VM, Shin J, et al. Comparison of endoscopic sinus surgery with and without image guidance. Am J Rhinol 2002;16(4):193–7.
11. Gibbons MD, Gunn CG, Niwas S, et al. Cost analysis of computer-aided endoscopic sinus surgery. Am J Rhinol 2001;15(2):71–5.
12. Javer AR, Genoway KA. Patient quality of life improvements with and without computer assistance in sinus surgery: outcomes study. J Otolaryngol 2006; 35(6):373–9.

13. Ramakrishnan VR, Orlandi RR, Citardi MJ, et al. The use of image-guided surgery in endoscopic sinus surgery: an evidence-based review with recommendations. Int Forum Allergy Rhinol 2013;3(3):236–41.

14. Sunkaraneni VS, Yeh D, Qian H, et al. Computer or not? Use of image guidance during endoscopic sinus surgery for chronic rhinosinusitis at St Paul's Hospital, Vancouver, and meta-analysis. J Laryngol Otol 2013;127(4):368–77.

15. Tabaee A, Hsu AK, Shrime MG, et al. Quality of life and complications following image-guided endoscopic sinus surgery. Otolaryngol Head Neck Surg 2006; 135(1):76–80.

16. Tschopp KP, Thomaser EG. Outcome of functional endonasal sinus surgery with and without CT-navigation. Rhinology 2008;46(2):116–20.

17. Metson R, Cosenza M, Gliklich RE, et al. The role of image-guidance systems for head and neck surgery. Arch Otolaryngol Head Neck Surg 1999;125(10):1100–4.

18. Kingdom TT, Orlandi RR. Image-guided surgery of the sinuses: current technology and applications. Otolaryngol Clin North Am 2004;37(2):381–400.

19. Smith TL, Stewart MG, Orlandi RR, et al. Indications for image-guided sinus surgery: the current evidence. Am J Rhinol 2007;21(1):80–3.

20. Surgery AAoO-HaN. Intraoperative use of computer-aided surgery. Available at: http://www.entnet.org/Practice/policyIntraOperativeSurgery.cfm. Accessed July 26, 2015.

21. Owen RG Jr, Kuhn FA. Supraorbital ethmoid cell. Otolaryngol Head Neck Surg 1997;116(2):254–61.

22. Chiu AG, Vaughan WC. Revision endoscopic frontal sinus surgery with surgical navigation. Otolaryngol Head Neck Surg 2004;130(3):312–8.

23. Anderson P, Sindwani R. Safety and efficacy of the endoscopic modified Lothrop procedure: a systematic review and meta-analysis. Laryngoscope 2009;119(9): 1828–33.

24. Draf W, Weber R, Keerl R, et al. Current aspects of frontal sinus surgery. I: endonasal frontal sinus drainage in inflammatory diseases of the paranasal sinuses. HNO 1995;43(6):352–7 [in German].

25. Chin D, Snidvongs K, Kalish L, et al. The outside-in approach to the modified endoscopic Lothrop procedure. Laryngoscope 2012;122(8):1661–9.

26. Yip JM, Seiberlin KA, Wormald PJ. Patient-reported olfactory function following endoscopic sinus surgery with modified endoscopic Lothrop procedure/Draf 3. Rhinology 2011;49(2):217–20.

27. Zacharek MA, Fong KJ, Hwang PH. Image-guided frontal trephination: a minimally invasive approach for hard-to-reach frontal sinus disease. Otolaryngol Head Neck Surg 2006;135(4):518–22.

28. Goode RL, Strelzow V, Fee WE Jr. Frontal sinus septectomy for chronic unilateral sinusitis. Otolaryngol Head Neck Surg 1980;88(1):18–21.

29. Sowerby LJ, MacNeil SD, Wright ED. Endoscopic frontal sinus septectomy in the treatment of unilateral frontal sinusitis: revisiting an open technique. J Otolaryngol Head Neck Surg 2009;38(6):652–4.

30. Bhavana K, Kumar R, Keshri A, et al. Minimally invasive technique for repairing CSF leaks due to defects of posterior table of frontal sinus. J Neurol Surg B Skull Base 2014;75(3):183–6.

31. Das PT, Balasubramanian D. External frontal sinusotomy and endoscopic repair of cerebrospinal fluid fistula in the posterior wall: preliminary report of a new technique. J Laryngol Otol 2011;125(8):802–6.

32. Hardy JM, Montgomery WW. Osteoplastic frontal sinusotomy: an analysis of 250 operations. Ann Otol Rhinol Laryngol 1976;85(4 Pt 1):523–32.

33. Weber R, Draf W, Keerl R, et al. Osteoplastic frontal sinus surgery with fat obliteration: technique and long-term results using magnetic resonance imaging in 82 operations. Laryngoscope 2000;110(6):1037–44.
34. Ansari K, Seikaly H, Elford G. Assessment of the accuracy and safety of the different methods used in mapping the frontal sinus. J Otolaryngol 2003;32(4): 254–8.
35. Fung MK. Template for frontal osteoplastic flap. Laryngoscope 1986;96(5):578–9.
36. Hybels RL. Transillumination during osteoplastic frontal sinusotomy. Laryngoscope 1981;91(9 Pt 1):1560.
37. Carrau RL, Snyderman CH, Curtin HB, et al. Computer-assisted frontal sinusotomy. Otolaryngol Head Neck Surg 1994;111(6):727–32.
38. Melroy CT, Dubin MG, Hardy SM, et al. Analysis of methods to assess frontal sinus extent in osteoplastic flap surgery: transillumination versus 6-ft Caldwell versus image guidance. Am J Rhinol 2006;20(1):77–83.
39. Sindwani R, Metson R. Impact of image guidance on complications during osteoplastic frontal sinus surgery. Otolaryngol Head Neck Surg 2004;131(3):150–5.

Standard Endoscopic Approaches in Frontal Sinus Surgery
Technical Pearls and Approach Selection

Zeina R. Korban, MD, Roy R. Casiano, MD*

KEYWORDS

- Frontal recess • Draf • Endoscopic modified Lothrop procedure (EMLP)
- Posterior frontal sinus wall

KEY POINTS

- Successful frontal sinus surgery relies on a complete frontal sinus surgery, and surgeons should approach management in a stepwise fashion from least invasive to advanced procedures depending on the case in hand and underlying pathophysiology.
- When performing a Draf III (EMLP), all intersinus septations need to be removed and a wide cavity created to facilitate postoperative medical therapy and improve symptoms.
- Maintaining dissection anterior to the coronal plane of the posterior frontal sinus wall prevents skull base injury.
- Before frontal sinus surgery, a complete anterior ethmoidectomy with identification of the fovea ethmoidalis and skeletonization of the medial orbital wall is necessary.
- Postoperative debridements and appropriate topical medical therapy are crucial in maintaining patency of the frontal drainage pathway.

 Video content accompanies this article at http://www.oto.theclinics.com.

INTRODUCTION

Frontal sinus surgery has always been considered a challenge. This is mainly attributed to its wide array of variable and complex anatomy, extent of disease, and associated scarring and osteoneogenesis that can ensue, either due to the primary disease process or previous incomplete surgery.[1] It is crucial to highlight that the mainstay of frontal sinus surgery for chronic rhinosinusitis, as it is with any of the sinuses, is to

The authors have nothing to disclose.
Department of Otolaryngology-Head & Neck Surgery, University of Miami, 1120 Northwest 14th Street, Miami, FL 33136, USA
* Corresponding author.
E-mail address: RCasiano@med.miami.edu

Otolaryngol Clin N Am 49 (2016) 989–1006
http://dx.doi.org/10.1016/j.otc.2016.03.022   oto.theclinics.com
0030-6665/16/$ – see front matter © 2016 Elsevier Inc. All rights reserved.

achieve and maintain an adequate frontal outflow tract (frontal recess and infundibulum) while preserving minimally diseased mucosal membranes where possible.[2] This has to be achieved by using a stepwise approach, identifying critical endoscopic anatomic landmarks, to minimize complications and obtain long-term good endoscopic surgical results.

In this article, we present the various endoscopic operative techniques and approaches to frontal sinus surgery in a systematized manner. We discuss the pertinence of useful anatomic landmarks to achieve safe frontal sinus surgery.

TREATMENT GOALS AND OUTCOMES

The most common causes of surgical failure are polyp recurrence, stenosis, and consequent scarring and/or osteoneogenesis.[3] This can be attributed, in part, to inadequate surgery, failure to recognize contributing anatomic barriers, and/or surgeon inexperience.

The goal is to relieve the patient's symptoms, restore functional mucociliary flow, achieve a wide frontal sinus ostium, and prevent long-term scarring and stenosis.

Multiple factors contribute to failure, and selecting the appropriate procedure for patients represents a challenge.

Mucociliary Flow

Messerklinger[4] first described frontal sinus ciliary flow. Knowledge of the ciliary flow pattern aids in successful frontal recess surgery. The cilia sweep up mucus along the interfrontal septum, laterally across the roof, medially along the floor toward the natural ostium. Mucosal preservation is fundamental when conceivable, although there are select situations in which this is impossible. Meticulous dissection and appropriate use of instrumentation and techniques aids in preventing unnecessary damage to normal mucosa while achieving one's goal of an adequate surgical ostium.

Osteoneogenesis

Controversies exist regarding the management of new bone formation in the region of the frontal sinus ostium. Some investigators advocate minimally invasive surgery with placement of stents and administration of oral and topical steroids in the postoperative period to prevent restenosis. The objective should be removal of the new bone to achieve a wide and adequate anteroposterior (AP) and lateral diameter, culture-directed postoperative antibiotics, office debridement, and close follow-up so as to intervene early in the event of symptomatic restenosis or closure of the frontal outflow tract. It is therefore very important to have proper visualization and instrumentation in the office setting to maximize the chances of a successful outcome.

PREOPERATIVE PLANNING

Before working in the region of the frontal sinus, it is imperative to have a robust conceptualization of the radiological anatomy and be conscious of the different anatomic relationships in this complex anatomic area. Being unfamiliar with the intricate anatomy of the inverted funnel, like frontal recess, predisposes to incomplete dissection and consequent failure with restenosis.[5]

The challenging location of the frontal sinus prompts anxiety for the surgeon because of the risk of injury to the anterior ethmoid artery, anterior cribriform plate, olfactory apparatus, and anterior skull base. Familiarizing oneself with a mental picture of the complex anatomy of the frontal recess and its surrounding cells gives the surgeon confidence in performing a safe surgery.

Once a decision for surgery has been made, a critical review of the axial, coronal, and sagittal cuts of the computed tomography (CT) scan must be performed.

Anatomy of the Frontal Recess

The frontal drainage outflow tract is bordered anteriorly by the posterior wall of the agger nasi or frontal infundibular cells, posteriorly by suprabullar air cells, laterally by the orbital roof, and medially by the vertical lamella of the middle turbinate (**Fig. 1**). The fovea ethmoidalis (ethmoid roof) forms the roof of the frontal recess. This is important to acknowledge, as it has been reported that the right fovea ethmoidalis slopes higher than the left in 59% of patients. Regardless of the asymmetries that may exist, it is more important to recognize this sloping for the potential of inadvertent penetration in the most medial aspect of the fovea ethmoidalis, particularly close to the insertion of the vertical lamella of the middle or superior turbinates, in the area corresponding to the lateral lamella of the cribriform plate. The depth of the olfactory fossa according to Keros[6] (type I: <3 mm, type II: 3–7 mm, type III: >7 mm) needs to be noted preoperatively and care should be taken when aggressively dissecting the medial fovea ethmoidalis, especially in patients with deeper olfactory fossae (type III Keros).[7] It is crucial to keep in mind that variable degrees of pneumatization may exist between patients, and from one side to the other. In addition, aplastic or hypoplastic frontal sinus cavities may be present.

Anatomic variants and cellular configurations along the frontal sinus outflow tract can contribute to obstruction and consequent disease. Having a clear understanding of the cells of the frontal sinus outflow tract leads to an appropriate initial approach to the frontal sinus.

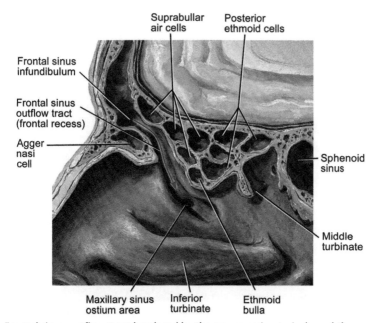

Fig. 1. Frontal sinus outflow tract bordered by the agger nasi anteriorly and the suprabullar cells posteriorly.

Agger Nasi

The agger nasi cell is the most anterior ethmoid air cell. It is located in the lateral nasal wall, anterior to the middle turbinate. It is found in 93% of the population and is best evaluated on coronal views.[8] It aids in understanding the transition from frontal recess to frontal sinus on coronal cuts of the preoperative CT scan. The superolateral attachment of the uncinate inserts into the inferior wall of the agger nasi cell. It also identifies the coronal plane leading superiorly to the frontal infundibular cells and frontal infundibulum (**Fig. 2**).

Intersinus Septal Cell

The intersinus septal cell represents pneumatization of the frontal sinus septum. It contributes to obstruction of the frontal recess and compromises the frontal ostium from a medial to lateral direction.[9,10] This cell needs to be addressed in frontal sinus surgery to ensure adequate lateral dimensions of the frontal sinus ostium to prevent subsequent closure or stenosis.

Frontal Ethmoidal Cells

The frontal infundibular cells border the frontal drainage outflow tract anteriorly approximately in the same coronal plane as the uncinate and agger nasi cell. These cells were previously described by Bent and Kuhn[11] into 4 types: type 1 (1 cell above the agger nasi), type II (2 or more cells above the agger nasi, but below the level of the frontal infundibulum and orbital roof), type III (at least 1 cell extending supraorbitally), and type IV (independent cell within the frontal sinus and not in contiguity with the other cells). They can be seen anywhere from 25% to 40% of the population and are located superior to the agger nasi cell.[10] The surgeon needs to be aware of the sequence of cells that are opened to ensure a wide and clear frontal recess without the crushing of these cells of the persistent of obstructive inflammatory disease of the frontal outflow tract. These cells are best evaluated on coronal and sagittal cuts (**Fig. 3**).

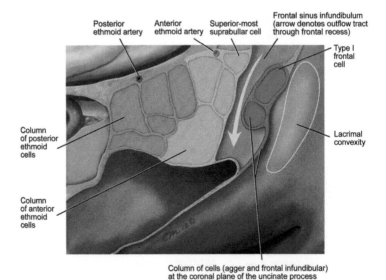

Fig. 2. Illustrating the relationship of the uncinate to the agger nasi cell.

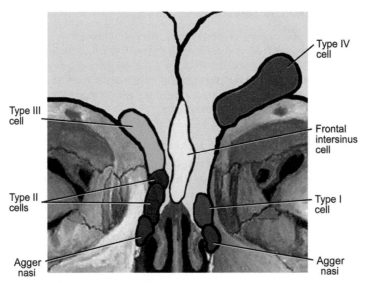

Type IV
cell

Type III
cell

Frontal
intersinus
cell

Type II
cells

Type I
cell

Agger
nasi

Agger
nasi

Fig. 3. Frontal recess cells.

Suprabullar Cell

The frontal outflow tract is bordered posteriorly by the suprabullar cells, best viewed on sagittal cuts. These cells lie above the ethmoid bulla and pneumatize up to its attachment to the skull base.[10] These cells may be variable in size and number, and do not enter the frontal sinus proper, unless the very last superior suprabullar cell pneumatizes superiorly, and extends into the frontal sinus (frontal bulla cell).

Frontal Bulla Cells

Frontal bulla cells are also best seen on sagittal views. They arise from the most superoanterior suprabullar cells. These cells pneumatize toward the frontal infundibulum along the skull base and posterior wall of the frontal sinus.[10]

The goal is to achieve a mental 3-dimensional reconstruction of the drainage pathway and associated cells so as to formulate an appropriate surgical plan. These cells vary among patients but their careful and methodical dissection is crucial to ensure a successful surgery.

Frontal Sinus Ostium

The frontal sinus ostium or infundibulum represents the narrowest point of the frontal sinus complex. The anteroposterior diameter of the frontal ostium needs to be assessed preoperatively. Patients who have a wide AP diameter will usually have an easier dissection and better postoperative prognosis. This is best assessed on sagittal cuts. Special care should be paid to patients with a narrow AP diameter, particularly in terms of mucosal preservation to prevent postoperative scarring and stenosis. This is particularly important in patients with no osteoneogenesis, where more advanced procedures may be needed, and mucosal sparing may not be possible. The goal is to achieve a wide AP diameter that can prevent consequent stenosis and scarring. In addition, evaluating the AP diameter preoperatively aids in reflecting the need for a drill out (Draf IIb or III) or more advanced procedures.

The surgeon should always gauge the degree of difficulty and keep in mind the possibility of extended procedures.

INDICATIONS FOR FRONTAL SINUSOTOMY

The most common indication for endoscopic frontal sinusotomy is chronic frontal sinusitis refractory to maximal medical management. This could be attributed to nasal polyposis, mucoceles, mechanical obstruction, osteoneogenesis, severe acute frontal sinusitis, benign and malignant neoplasms, and frontal sinus fractures, among others.

The aim is to achieve functional mucus clearance with removal of all frontal recess cells and prevent future restenosis and scarring.[12]

PATIENT POSITIONING

Before starting any endoscopic sinus surgery, proper patient positioning should be ensured. The patient should be placed in a supine position on the operating table with the table tilted to 30° anti-Trendelenburg to prevent venous congestion and allow more adequate control of hemostasis intraoperatively. The head should be in a neutral position to allow the surgeon to work in a plane parallel to the skull base and prevent inadvertent injury. The surgeon typically stands on the right side of the patient. The video tower and associated imaging devices are positioned at the head of the table facing the surgeon.

Both eyes need to be protected with a clear adhesive dressing, to be able to detect acute proptosis or chemosis, consistent with an orbital injury or hematoma. The eyes should be periodically palpated during the superior ethmoidectomy and frontal sinusotomy. The forehead, eyes, nose, and upper lip need to be exposed.

We advocate the use of a 30-degree, 45-degree, and/or 70-degree scope in frontal sinus surgery. The endoscopes and instruments should never cross. Using angled scopes facilitates easier passage of instruments and better visualization.

It is important to operate in a comfortable setting.

KEY LANDMARKS

The key to safe frontal sinus surgery is accurate knowledge of anatomy. We advocate the use of several key anatomic landmarks to warrant safe endoscopic frontal sinus surgery.

Key landmarks described by Dr Casiano in 2001 include the following[12]:

- Uncinate process superior attachment
- Middle turbinate vertical lamella
- Vertical line from the maxillary natural ostium area, parallel to the nasolacrimal apparatus convexity
- Anterior ethmoid artery
- The suprabullar and agger nasi cells
- Frontal sinus posterior wall.

Identifying the frontal sinus outflow tract is the initial and most fundamental step in frontal sinus surgery. Before addressing the frontal recess, an ethmoidectomy should be achieved to allow for safe frontal sinus surgery with a clear identification of the fovea ethmoidalis.[5]

Skeletonization of the medial orbital wall (lamina papyracea) needs to be achieved to ensure adequate dissection and exposure of the frontal sinus.

The frontal recess should be addressed in a posterior to anterior and a medial to lateral direction to avoid skull base penetration, particularly at the level of the lateral lamella of the cribriform plate. It can be initially identified approximately 5 to 10 mm behind the anterior attachment of the middle turbinate. We advocate using the ball probe initially to prevent inadvertent skull base injury. The correct point of entry will be superomedially, adjacent to the vertical lamella of the middle turbinate, and posterior to the coronal plane of the superior attachment of the uncinate process, or anterior to the coronal plane of the face of the ethmoid bulla if intact. The tip of the probe should be directed superolaterally, without exerting pressure (2-finger palpation), and toward the direction of the orbital roof and parallel to the sloping fovea ethmoidalis.

The location of the anterior ethmoid artery always should be kept in mind. It is located an average of 20 mm from the anterior attachment of the middle turbinate or 10 mm from the posterior wall of the frontal sinus. All septations should be displaced anteroinferiorly at the level of the anterior ethmoid artery to avoid inadvertent injury. If there is to be aggressive manipulation in the area, it is best to perform this medially, so as to minimize orbital retraction of the artery if severed close to the orbital wall near the entry into its canal.

We recommend using the 70-degree telescope especially when internal frontal sinus manipulation is indicated.

The posterior wall of the frontal sinus serves as a guide during surgery to avoid intracranial penetration and injury at the level of the cribriform plate. This will be discussed later in this article.[12]

We also advocate the use of the frontal probe, giraffe forceps, and an angled microdebrider to remove the frontal recess cell septations, while preserving normal mucosa circumferentially at the level of the infundibulum. Small septations should be carefully removed with overlying mucosa, without stripping of infundibular mucosa, or crushing of septations and mucosal elements, obliterating the frontal outflow tract.

Care should be taken with using the microdebrider and it entails surgeon experience. It should be used only to clean up loose mucosal edges and not for meticulous dissection in narrow passages. The opening of the angled microdebrider should initially be pointed anteriorly, until the posterior wall of the frontal and anterior ethmoid artery has been identified. The tip should always be kept moving, and never kept in a stationary location, to minimize inadvertent bone and mucosal removal, and orbital or skull base penetration. It also never should be pointed toward the orbit, until the orbit has been clearly identified.

FRONTAL SINUS PROCEDURES

The endoscopic endonasal approach to the frontal sinus has become the standard of care in chronic rhinosinusitis recalcitrant to medical management. This is attributed to a greater understanding of chronic inflammatory disease affecting the sinuses and sinus pathophysiology. Additionally, surgical experience with endoscopic instrumentation has improved and become more widespread in the past couple of decades.[13]

Diverse endonasal sinusotomy and drainage options have been established depending on the extent of dissection required. These are based on the Draf system classification.

Draf Type I Frontal Sinusotomy

Type I frontal sinusotomy encompasses drainage of the frontal recess without major frontal sinus disease. It entails removal of the anterosuperior ethmoidal cells obstructing the frontal sinus outflow tract and serves to expose the frontal ostium. The roof of the agger nasi (or most superior frontal infundibular cell) is left intact. Mucosa of the outflow tract is circumferentially preserved.

This represents the least-invasive frontal sinus procedure with removal of disease, inferior to the frontal ostium. It is not frequently used, especially when frontal sinus pathology is present (**Fig. 4**).

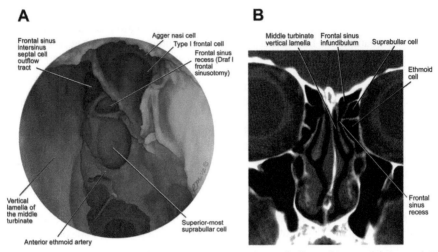

Fig. 4. (A) Draf I, with the roof of the agger nasi and suprabullar cell intact. (B) Coronal CT view depicting area of dissection in a Draf I. *Red dotted line* represents the area of dissection in a Draf I. Keeping the roof of the agger nasi and suprabullar cell intact.

Draf Type II Frontal Sinusotomy

Draf IIA

In a Draf IIA, the frontal sinus is opened between the middle turbinate medially and the lamina papyracea laterally with a larger opening of the frontal sinus floor. It entails clear exposure of the internal frontal sinus cavity and removal of all ethmoidal cells protruding into the frontal sinus 8. The roof of the agger nasi cell and the (superior-most) suprabullar cell is removed until a maximum AP diameter of the frontal neo-ostium is attained. Typically, this could be anywhere from 6 to 8 mm without significant osteoneogenesis. Care is taken to preserve mucosa and maintain a plane anterior to the posterior wall of the frontal sinus (**Fig. 5**).

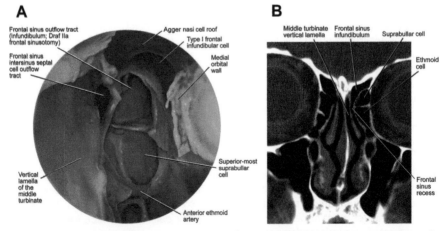

Fig. 5. (A) Draf IIa illustrating clear exposure of the internal frontal sinus cavity from the lamina papyracea to the vertical lamella of the middle turbinate. (B) Coronal CT view depicting the area of dissection in a Draf IIa. *Red dotted line* represents the extent of dissection in a Draf IIa. Depict removal of the roof of the agger nasi cell and suprabullar cell.

A Type IIA frontal sinusotomy is recommended in patients with frontal sinus pathology, failed type I frontal sinusotomy, and frontal sinuses with a large anteroposterior diameter, and a broad ethmoid, whereby removal of the ethmoidal cells will yield a wide drainage outflow tract.[14]

ADVANCED FRONTAL SINUS PROCEDURES

In the past, recalcitrant frontal sinusitis was managed through external procedures and frontal sinus obliteration with harvesting of an osteoplastic flap. This entailed a high failure and complication rate. Cerebrospinal fluid leaks, mucocele formation, frontal bossing, cosmetic defects, and chronic pain syndromes were among the many complications that ensued.[15]

In recent years, extended endoscopic frontal sinusotomy procedures (Draf IIb or III) have been described and have replaced the previous open and obliteration techniques.[16]

Extended frontal sinusotomy procedures may be indicated in chronic frontal rhinosinusitis refractory to medical and surgical traditional endoscopic management. In some cases, primary advanced procedures are indicated, particularly when dealing with a narrow AP diameter.

Other indications include the following:

- Patients with chronic frontal sinusitis and significant comorbidities: cystic fibrosis, aspirin-exacerbated respiratory disease, ciliary dysfunction disorders
- Allergic fungal rhinosinusitis
- Inverted papilloma
- Failed previous conservative surgery
- Extensive scarring
- Mucocele
- Osteoneogenesis
- Recurrent polyposis with focal disease limited mainly to the frontal and anterior ethmoid sinus cavities

Patient selection for advanced procedures is not clear-cut. Cases should be individualized, taking into account the potential for future stenosis and scarring. The goal is symptom relief while reducing the need for further revision surgeries. Achieving a wide, patent frontal sinus, even with a primary endoscopic modified Lothrop procedure (EMLP), should be the goal.

A Draf IIb procedure consists of removal of the frontal sinus floor between the lamina papyracea and the nasal septum.[16]

A Draf III is a median drainage procedure that entails removing the upper part of the nasal septum and the frontal sinus septations to achieve a maximal possible opening.

This procedure, now known as the EMLP, is based on an original technique proposed by Lothrop in 1914,[17] whereby removal of the frontal sinus floor was achieved through an external ethmoidectomy bilaterally.

The endoscopic modification entails the absence of this external incision (Video 1).

Key landmarks that should be kept in mind during advanced frontal sinusotomy procedures include the following:

- Anterior one-fourth of the vertical lamella of the middle turbinate anterior to the coronal plane of the posterior frontal wall (medial wall of the frontal infundibulum)
- Anterior olfactory cleft and cribriform plate, and olfactory fibrils
- Posterior wall of the frontal sinus
- Superior perpendicular plate

After skeletonizing the medial orbital wall and anterior ethmoid roof, the posterior frontal sinus wall in its coronal plane can be identified, at least on one side.

This can be achieved either through a unilateral frontal infundibulum, or if the infundibulum is significantly fibrotic or ossified, and difficult to safely identify, a supraturbinal or transeptal approach can be performed more anteriorly and in the midline.

Care should be taken during a transeptal approach, particularly in patients with a narrow AP diameter, as this can put the patient at risk for a cerebrospinal fluid leak and skull base injury (**Fig. 6**). Intraoperative navigation may be useful in these approaches, until significant experience is acquired.

For a Draf IIb, if one frontal infundibulum is identified, the anterior one-fourth of the middle turbinate vertical lamella is removed, heading in the direction of the posterior wall of frontal infundibulum, where the vertical lamella inserts into the medial bony wall of the infundibulum. Next, the anterior cribriform plate is identified inferomedial to the posterior wall of the frontal infundibulum, medial to the middle turbinate vertical lamella, but posterior to the coronal plane of the posterior wall of the frontal infundibulum. The junction of the perpendicular plate with the frontal intersinus septum is identified by removal the bony medial wall of the frontal infundibulum, where the middle turbinate attached. This can be done with angled C-spine curettes or a cutting bur on an irrigating angled microdebrider handpiece. Care is warranted in preserving the mucosa of the posterior wall of the frontal recess whenever deemed possible or feasible (**Figs. 7** and **8**).

In certain cases, particularly in unilateral lesions, presence of intersinus cells, or suprabullar cells with significant supraorbital and lateral extension, the Draf IIb can be extended.[18] This can be achieved either by removal of either the frontal intersinus

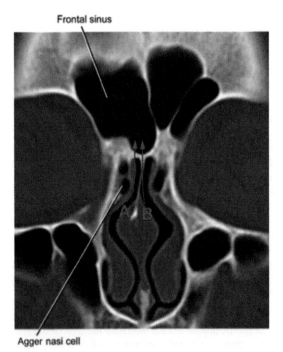

Fig. 6. Supraturbinal (A) and transeptal approach (B) at the coronal plane of the anterior middle turbinate attachment, bypassing the frontal recess area.

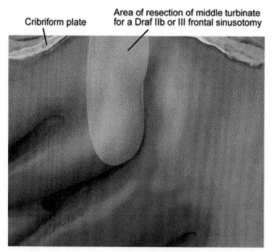

Fig. 7. Illustrating the area of resection of the middle turbinate.

septum, or the anterosuperior nasal septum. This attains a wide exposure without damage to the contralateral frontal sinus drainage. The nasal septectomy can be created more inferior and posterior to gain access to the supraorbital cells.[18] However, care must be taken not to extend the septectomy posteriorly to the coronal plane of the anterior cribriform plate.

In many situations, significant fibrosis and osteoneogenesis can be seen in the area of the frontal infundibulum, and to achieve a wide frontal cavity and prevent future stenosis, a Draf III (EMLP, frontal sinus drill out) is warranted.[19]

To proceed, the anterosuperior perpendicular plate of the ethmoid is resected, either with cutting forceps or powered instrumentation, to achieve an anterosuperior septectomy. An orientation anterior to the coronal plane of the posterior wall of the frontal sinus, as seen through the frontal sinus ostium or through a transeptal frontal sinusotomy, should be maintained. This avoids inadvertent intracranial penetration

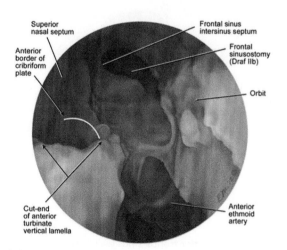

Fig. 8. Junction of the perpendicular plate with the frontal intersinus septum.

or injury to the olfactory apparatus at the level of the cribriform, or more inferiorly over the olfactory mucosa of the nasal septum or vertical lamella or the middle and superior turbinates (**Fig. 9**).

This also aids in facilitating exposure and bi-nostril introduction of instrumentation.

Working simultaneously from both sides of the nose, the perpendicular plate is followed superiorly toward the intersinus frontal septum, anterior to the plane that was previously discussed. The thick, dense bone at the nasofrontal "beak" area is reduced either with cervical spine bone curettes, or an aggressive 60-degree cutting burr until clear visualization of the posterior wall of the frontal sinus is achieved. Once a common frontal sinus ostium is achieved, enlargement is resumed using a combination of microdebrider blades and drills, to achieve a wide horseshoe opening, extending orbit to orbit, and posterior frontal table to nasion. The nasion dermis can be intentionally identified as a marker for the anterior limit of dissection. The medial supracanthal skin region could serve as a landmark for the lateral limits of dissection. This dermis is found laterally, as one drills the common frontal, anterior to the coronal plane of the posterior frontal wall. The lateral recesses of the frontal sinus should be visualized bilaterally and irrigated of any debris or mucin. All interfrontal cells and septations should be effectively removed (**Figs. 10 and 11**).

The final common frontal cavity should measure approximately, 8 to 10 mm anteroposteriorly (at the nasofrontal beak area) and 20 to 26 mm from orbital wall to orbital wall[15] (**Figs. 12 and 13**).

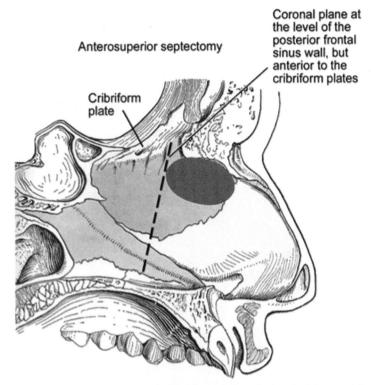

Fig. 9. Vertical line from the posterior frontal sinus wall to the level of the nasal floor anterior to the cribriform plate representing a safe area of dissection.

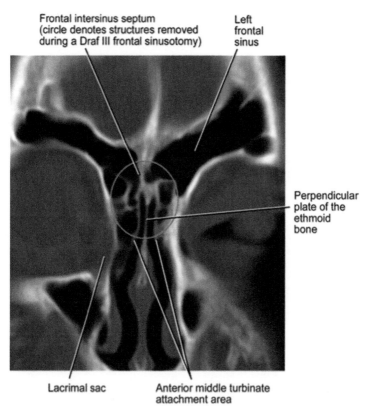

Frontal intersinus septum
(circle denotes structures removed
during a Draf III frontal sinusotomy)

Left
frontal
sinus

Perpendicular
plate of the
ethmoid
bone

Lacrimal sac

Anterior middle turbinate
attachment area

Fig. 10. Coronal image denoting the perpendicular plate of the ethmoid and intersinus septum that needs to be removed in an EMLP.

It is imperative to create the largest possible opening. The size of the common frontal cavity attained is one of the main factors that contributes to future stenosis, despite associated fungal sinusitis and nasal polyposis.[20] In a study performed on 80 modified endoscopic lothrop (MEL) patients, narrowing typically occurs in the first 12 months after surgery and remains stable after that.[20,21] It narrows to approximately less than half of the original intraoperative opening in approximately one-third of the patients, and complete closure may be seen in approximately 10% of the patients.[15] However, not all are symptomatic or require fairly effective endoscopic revision surgery. Patency, as defined by a greater than 50% of the original intraoperative opening size, is achieved in more than 67% of the patients.

COMBINED ABOVE AND BELOW TECHNIQUE

Utilization of combined endoscopic with limited external incisions may be indicated in select cases. This may involve limited transverse forehead crease, superior lid, lateral brow, or a more formal bicoronal incision. Combined approaches may be necessary to maximize visualization and introduction of instrumentation, to safely access the cavity and facilitate dissection. The presence of a type IV frontal cell obstructing the frontal drainage, that cannot be accessed endoscopically, may warrant a combined technique, as well as certain bony neoplasms, or lesions involving

Frontal intersinus septum
(circle denotes what is removed
during a Draf III frontal sinusotomy)

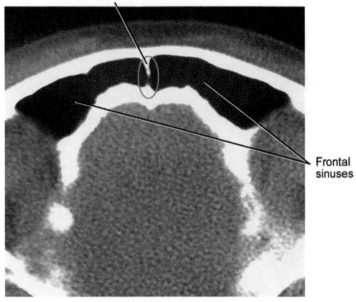

Frontal
sinuses

Fig. 11. Axial images before an EMLP.

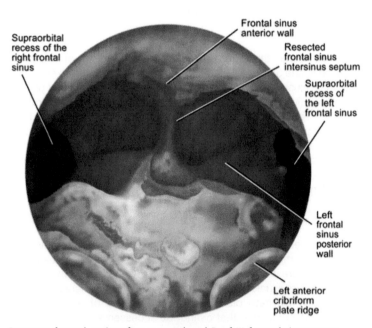

Fig. 12. Common frontal cavity after a completed Draf III frontal sinusotomy.

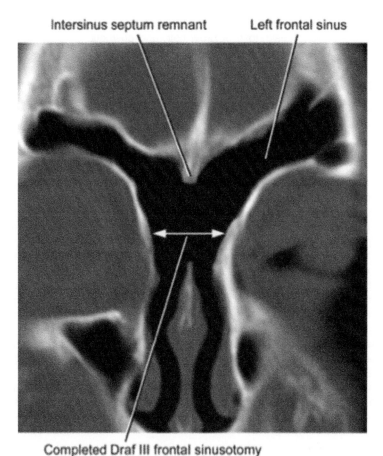

Fig. 13. A coronal CT illustrating a completed Draf III frontal sinusotomy.

the lateral recess of the frontal sinus supraorbitally, such as inverted papillomas or mucoceles.

Combined techniques also may be required for adequate and safe margins in oncological resection of other malignant of benign neoplasms.

These techniques also may be used to establish frontal sinus drainage when no pathway can be achieved endoscopically.

Frontal Sinus Trephination

A frontal sinus trephination is not commonly used any more. However, in select cases, it may be useful to temporarily decompress a mucopyocele or for introduction of telescopes or dye material into the frontal sinus. Following the endoscopic identification of the frontal recess, the medial brow incision is placed. The location usually depends on the underlying pathology, particularly when a mucocele is present.[22] The incision is generally placed parallel to the hair follicles and medial to the supratrochlear nerve. The incision is carried down to the anterior table. A small burr is used to enter the sinus. Intraoperative navigation can be used, but is usually not necessary. The general tenet is to perform a bone window into the frontal sinus that is limited to 5 mm.

Complications may include damage to the supratrochlear and supraorbital nerves with secondary hypesthesia, loss of brow hair, and cosmetic deformity secondary to the incision.[22,23]

POSTOPERATIVE CARE

Postoperative management is aimed at maintaining patency of the frontal sinus cavity. Nasal saline irrigations and postoperative debridements are essential in minimizing postoperative wound infections, granulation overgrowth, and potential restenosis or closure of the frontal sinus outflow tract, especially in patients who had significant mucosa and bone removal (Draf IIb and III).

Patients should present for their first postoperative debridement 7 to 10 days after surgery for removal of crusts and inflamed tissue, and to reduce local inflammation and consequent infection. They are then seen approximately 1 month later. After their second postoperative visit, further follow-ups and debridements are individualized depending on the specific needs of the patients. Long-term follow-up relies on the underlying pathophysiology and is based on the patency of the sinus outflow tracts and control of their sinonasal inflammation with medical therapy.

Use of culture-directed topical and oral antibiotic therapy and topical and systemic steroid administration depends on the underlying pathophysiology and postoperative wound healing.

Some investigators advocate the use of stents, placed intraoperatively, to prevent future stenosis and promote mucosalization. Controversy exists and no standardized indications are available, however. Stents may be considered for narrow neo-ostiums, and circumferential exposure of bone.

However, granulation tissue formation, biofilm production, and crusting can ensue from the use of stents.[24] In-office management of symptomatic, stenotic ostia also may be necessary but using a variety of instrumentation, including balloon sinuplasty.

LITERATURE REVIEW

Outcomes of the previously described endoscopic frontal sinus approaches vary in the literature. This mainly depends on patient selection and the indication for the procedure. It is difficult to compare outcomes, particularly due to different surgical techniques and classification of patency and stenosis.

Various studies exist that support advanced frontal sinus procedures. **Table 1** summarizes various investigators' results after performing an EMLP, in terms of patency

| Table 1 | | | | |
| Outcomes of endoscopic modified Lothrop procedures (EMLP) | | | | |
Author	Patients	Mean Follow-up (mo)	Patency[a] (%)	Symptoms (%)
Becker et al,[25] 1995	14	9	100	14
Casiano & Livingston,[15] 1998	21	24	57	21
Wormald,[26] 2003	83	21.9	93	25
Shirazi et al,[27] 2007	97	18	77	23
Anderson & Sindwani,[28] 2009	612	28.5	95.9	16
Wormald et al,[29] 2014	229	45	95	5

[a] % Patency defined as a visible frontal sinus ostium.
Data from Refs.[15,25–29]

and persistence of symptoms after follow-up. Results are dependent on a mixed population with chronic frontal rhinosinusitis as the common indication.

SUMMARY

Endoscopic surgery of the frontal sinus and its outflow tract remains one of the most difficult endoscopic techniques. The goals of a successful frontal sinus surgery are to achieve long-term patency, avoid revision surgery, and minimize symptoms and complications. The indicated frontal sinus procedure is tailored to the patient's underlying pathology and anatomy. Being familiar with the radiological and endoscopic anatomy enables surgeons to provide adequate treatment for their patients, keeping in mind key landmarks can aid in accurate and safe surgery. Performing and mastering advanced frontal sinus techniques has been an increasing trend and should be advocated when necessary.

SUPPLEMENTARY DATA

Supplementary data related to this article can be found at http://dx.doi.org/10.1016/j.otc.2016.03.022.

REFERENCES

1. Wormald PJ. Surgical approach to the frontal sinus and frontal recess. Endoscopic sinus surgery. 3rd edition. Chapter 7. New York: Thieme; 2012. p. 81–102.
2. Shaefer SD, Close LG. Endoscopic management of frontal sinus disease. Laryngoscope 1990;100:155–60.
3. Bassiouni A, Wormald PJ. Role of frontal sinus surgery in nasal polyp recurrence. Laryngoscope 2013;123(1):36–41.
4. Messerklinger W. On the drainage of the normal frontal sinus of man. Acta Otolaryngol 1967;63(2):176–81.
5. Schaefer SD. Modern concepts of frontal sinus surgery. Laryngoscope 2001;111: 137–46.
6. Keros P. Uber die praktische Bedeutung der Niveauunterschiede de lamina cribrosa des Ethmoids. Laryngol Rhinol Otol (Stuttg) 1965;41:808–13.
7. Floreani SR, Nair SB, Switajewski MC, et al. Endoscopic anterior ethmoidal artery ligation: a cadaver study. Laryngoscope 2006;116(7):1263–7.
8. Bolger WE, Butzin CA, Parsons DS. Paranasal sinus bony anatomic variations and mucosal abnormalities: CT analysis for endoscopic sinus surgery. Laryngoscope 1991;101(1 Pt 1):56–64.
9. Wormald PJ. Anatomy of the frontal recess and frontal sinus with three-dimensional reconstruction. Chapter 6. New York: Thieme; 2012. p. 45–6.
10. Chiu AG, Adappa ND, Reed J, et al. Frontal sinusotomy: Chapter 11; Atlas of endoscopic sinus and skull Base Surgery. Elsevier Health Sciences; 2012. p. 93–4.
11. Bent JP, Cuilty-Siller C, Kuhn FA. The frontal cell as a cause of frontal sinus obstruction. American Journal of Rhinology 1994;8:185–91.
12. Casiano RR. Endoscopic sinonasal dissection guide. Chapter 5. New York: Thieme; 2012. p. 54–5.
13. Casiano RR. A stepwise surgical technique using the medial orbital floor as the key landmark in performing endoscopic sinus surgery. Laryngoscope 2001; 111(6):964–74.

14. Stammberger H. Endoscopic diagnosis and surgery of the paranasal sinuses and anterior skull base-the Messerklinger technique and advanced applications from the Graz School. Tuttlingen (Germany): Storz GmbH; 1998.
15. Casiano RR, Livingston JA. Endoscopic Lothrop procedure: the University of Miami experience. Am J Rhinol 1998;12(5):335–9.
16. Draf W. Endonasal micro-endoscopic frontal sinus surgery, the Fulda concept. Operat Tech Otolaryngol Head Neck Surg 1991;2:234–40.
17. Lothrop HA. XIV. Frontal Sinus suppuration: the establishment of permanent nasal drainage; the closure of external fistulae; epidermization of sinus. Ann Surg 1914; 59(6):937–57.
18. Eloy JA, Friedel ME, Murray KP, et al. Modified hemi-Lothrop procedure for supra-orbital frontal sinus access: a cadaveric feasibility study. Otolaryngol Head Neck Surg 2011;145(3):489–93.
19. Casiano RR. Endoscopic sinonasal dissection guide. Chapter 6. New York: Thieme; 2012. p. 54–5.
20. Tran K, Buele A, Singhal D, et al. Frontal ostium restenosis after the endoscopic modified Lothrop procedure. Laryngoscope 2007;117(8):1457–62.
21. Rajapaska SP, Ananda A, Cain TM, et al. Frontal ostium neo-osteogenesis and restenosis after modified endoscopic Lothrop procedure in an animal model. Clin Otolaryngol Allied Sci 2004;29(4):386–8.
22. Bednarski KA, Senior BA. Advanced frontal surgery techniques. Chapter 28; Rhinology – diseases of the nose, sinuses and skull base. New York: Thieme; 2012. p. 361–9.
23. Batra PS, Citardi MJ, Lanza DC. Combined endoscopic trephination and endoscopic frontal sinusotomy for management of complex frontal sinus pathology. Am J Rhinol 2005;19(5):435–41.
24. Maeso PA, Das S, Kountakis SE. Revision endoscopic frontal sinus surgery. Chapter 15; Revision sinus surgery. Springer; 2008. p. 132.
25. Becker DG, Moore D, Lindsey WH, et al. Modified transnasal endoscopic Lothrop procedure: further considerations. Laryngoscope 1995;105(11):1161–6.
26. Wormald PJ. Salvage frontal sinus surgery: the endoscopic modified Lothrop procedure. Laryngoscope 2003;113(2):276–83.
27. Shirazi MA, Silver AL, Stankiewicz JA. Surgical outcomes following the endoscopic modified Lothrop procedure. Laryngoscope 2007;117(5):765–9.
28. Anderson P, Sindwani R. Safety and efficacy of the endoscopic modified Lothrop procedure: a systematic review and meta-analysis. Laryngoscope 2009;119(9): 1828–33.
29. Wormald PJ, Naidoo Y, Bassiouni A, et al. Long-term outcomes for the endoscopic modified Lothrop/Draf III procedure: a 10-year review. Laryngoscope 2014;124(1):43–9.

Endoscopic Approaches to the Frontal Sinus

Modifications of the Existing Techniques and Proposed Classification

Jean Anderson Eloy, MD[a,b,c,d,]*, Alejandro Vázquez, MD[a],
James K. Liu, MD[a,b,c], Soly Baredes, MD[a,b]

KEYWORDS

- Frontal sinus • Frontal sinusotomy • Endoscopic modified Lothrop procedure
- Lothrop procedure • Modified hemi-Lothrop procedure
- Modified mini-Lothrop procedure • Modified subtotal-Lothrop procedure
- Extended Draf IIB

KEY POINTS

- The modified hemi-Lothrop procedure (Eloy IIC) involves an ipsilateral Draf IIB and an anterosuperior septectomy window for access to the lateral recess of the ipsilateral frontal sinus via the contralateral nasal cavity.
- The modified mini-Lothrop procedure (Eloy IID) involves a contralateral Draf IIB and a frontal intersinus septectomy.
- The modified subtotal-Lothrop procedure (Eloy IIE) involves an ipsilateral Draf IIB with a superior septectomy and frontal intersinus septectomy.

Continued

Financial Disclosures: None.
Conflicts of Interest: None.
Presented in Part at the 59th Annual Meeting of the American Rhinologic Society, Vancouver, BC, September 28, 2013.
[a] Department of Otolaryngology – Head and Neck Surgery, Rutgers New Jersey Medical School, Newark, NJ, USA; [b] Center for Skull Base and Pituitary Surgery, Neurological Institute of New Jersey, Rutgers New Jersey Medical School, Newark, NJ, USA; [c] Department of Neurological Surgery, Rutgers New Jersey Medical School, Newark, NJ, USA; [d] Department of Ophthalmology and Visual Science, Rutgers New Jersey Medical School, 90 Bergen Street, Suite 8100, Newark, NJ 07103, USA
* Corresponding author. Rhinology and Sinus Surgery, Otolaryngology Research, Endoscopic Skull Base Surgery Program, Department of Otolaryngology – Head and Neck Surgery, Neurological Institute of New Jersey, Rutgers New Jersey Medical School, 90 Bergen Street, Suite 8100, Newark, NJ 07103.
E-mail address: jean.anderson.eloy@gmail.com

Continued

- The modified central-Lothrop procedure (Eloy IIF) involves resection of the frontal sinus floor bilaterally, with a superior septectomy and frontal intersinus septectomy, while preserving both frontal sinus recesses.
- These alterations represent expansion on the current Draf or nasofrontal classification systems and approaches.

 Video content accompanies this article at http://www.oto.theclinics.com.

INTRODUCTION

The frontal sinus has proven to be anatomically challenging, both with respect to surgical access and management of chronic and recurrent disease. There exist numerous anatomic variations between patients and even between sides in the same patient.[1] Treatments of frontal sinus disease range from conservative long-term medical management to aggressive open surgical procedures. Advances in frontal sinus surgery have allowed for movement away from the more invasive and potentially disfiguring open approaches to less aggressive, endonasal approaches.

The Lothrop procedure described in 1914 consisted of an intranasal ethmoidectomy followed by an external Lynch-type approach with resection of the medial frontal sinus floor, superior nasal septum, and intersinus septum, which created a large frontonasal communication. The microendoscopic and endoscopic modifications to Lothrop's original technique have been described in the literature, notably by Draf,[2] Gross and colleagues,[3] and Close and colleagues.[4] These investigators have detailed an endonasal approach similar in concept to Lothrop that also involves creating a large common drainage pathway between the paired frontal sinuses. Efforts to reduce invasiveness and preserve the natural architecture of the frontal sinus have led recently to the description of the modified hemi-Lothrop procedure,[5–8] the modified mini-Lothrop procedure,[9,10] and the modified subtotal-Lothrop procedure.[11,12]

DISCUSSION OF TECHNIQUES

Current and common methods of classification for endonasal frontal sinus drainage techniques include the Draf and nasofrontal approaches.[13] The recent modifications of endonasal frontal sinus techniques are not included within these classification systems. For this reason, a new classification system consolidating the 2 previous methods and allowing for inclusion of the 3 recently published modifications (as well as a new modification) has been designed (**Table 1**). This article discusses these modifications in the context of the new classification scheme.

Standard Frontal Sinus Approaches

Draf I (nasofrontal approach I or Eloy I): This procedure consists of an anterior ethmoidectomy for drainage of the frontal sinus recess without dissection of the frontal sinus outflow pathway (**Fig. 1**A). This involves removal of obstructing disease inferior to the frontal sinus recess. In this technique, the anterosuperior ethmoidal cells (including the agger nasi) are resected without disrupting the frontal sinus outflow pathway.

Draf IIA (nasofrontal approach II or Eloy IIA): This procedure entails the removal of the anterior ethmoidal cells and frontal cells protruding into the frontal sinus outflow pathway, creating an opening between the middle turbinate medially and the lamina

Table 1
Classification schemes of endoscopic approaches to the frontal sinus

Draf	Nasofrontal Approach	Eloy's Proposed Modifications	Description
I	I	I	Anterior ethmoidectomy with drainage of the frontal sinus recess without touching the frontal sinus outflow pathway
IIA	II	IIA	Removal of the anterior ethmoidal cells and frontal cells protruding into the frontal sinus outflow pathway creating an opening between the middle turbinate medially and the lamina papyracea laterally
IIB	III	IIB	Removal of the frontal sinus floor between the nasal septum medially and the lamina papyracea laterally
		IIC	Ipsilateral removal of the frontal sinus floor between the nasal septum medially and the lamina papyracea laterally; superior septectomy for access from the contraletaral side and enhanced access to the lateral supraorbital frontal sinus and supraorbital ethmoid regions. This also provides binostril, bimanual manipulation; previously described as a modified hemi-Lothrop procedure.
		IID	Contralateral removal of the frontal sinus floor between the nasal septum medially and the lamina papyracea laterally with addition of an intersinus septectomy for drainage of the diseased frontal sinus to the contralateral recess; previously described as a modified mini-Lothrop procedure
		IIE	Ipsilateral removal of the frontal sinus floor between the nasal septum medially and the lamina papyracea laterally; superior septectomy for access from the contraletaral side and enhanced access to the lateral supraorbital frontal sinus and supraorbital ethmoid regions; intersinus septectomy for access to the entire posterior wall of the frontal sinus; preservation of the contralateral frontal sinus recess; previously described as a modified subtotal-Lothrop procedure
		IIF	Central resection of the frontal sinus floor bilaterally, with a superior septectomy and frontal intersinus septectomy, while preserving both frontal sinus recesses; also termed a modified central-Lothrop procedure
III	IV	III	Bilateral removal of the floor of the frontal sinus anterior to the middle turbinates from 1 lamina papyracea to the next with superior septectomy and intersinus septectomy; also termed a modified Lothrop procedure

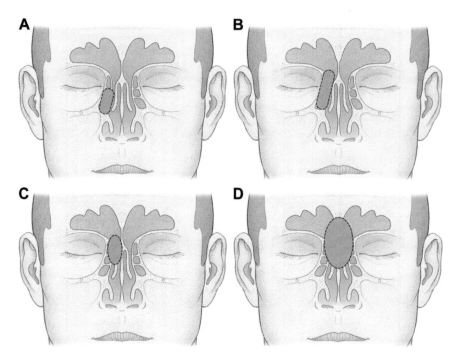

Fig. 1. Artwork in the coronal plane depicting (*A*) Draf I, (*B*) Draf IIA, (*C*) Draf IIB, and (*D*) Draf III procedures. Area containing the resected structures is depicted with the red outline. (© 2015 Chris Gralapp, Fairfax, CA.)

papyracea laterally (**Fig. 1**B). This in turn leads to enlargement of the frontal sinus outflow pathway.

Draf IIB (nasofrontal approach III or Eloy IIB): This procedure also enlarges the frontal sinus outflow pathway and consists of the removal of the frontal sinus floor between the nasal septum medially and the lamina papyracea laterally (**Fig. 1**C). The goal of this procedure is to achieve maximal opening of the frontal sinus outflow pathway on 1 side.

Draf III (nasofrontal approach IV or Eloy III): In this procedure, bilateral removal of the floor of the frontal sinus anterior to the middle turbinates from 1 lamina papyracea to the next is performed, with a superior septectomy and intersinus septectomy; this is also termed a modified Lothrop procedure (**Fig. 1**D). With this procedure, a contiguous bilateral enlargement of the frontal sinus drainage pathway is achieved.

Modified Hemi-Lothrop Procedure (Eloy IIC)

The modified hemi-Lothrop procedure (Eloy IIC) has previously been described as a technique used to improve access to the lateral recess (supraorbital extension) of an affected frontal sinus or supraorbital ethmoid cell (**Fig. 2**).[5–7] The procedure combines an ipsilateral Draf IIB (removal of the frontal sinus floor from the nasal septum medially to the lamina papyracea laterally) and a superior septectomy. The superior septectomy window allows insertion of an endoscope and instruments via the contralateral side, thus providing greater access and visualization of the lateral frontal sinus recess of the affected ipsilateral frontal sinus or supraorbital ethmoid. This technique also provides for binostril and bimanual instrumentation (**Fig. 3**). The ability to perform

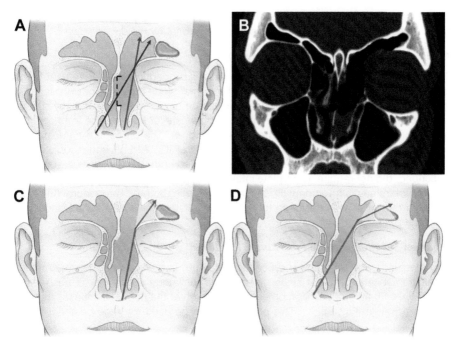

Fig. 2. (*A*) Artwork in the coronal plane showing the approach to the contralateral frontal sinus with Eloy IIC procedure, also known as the modified hemi-Lothrop procedure. (*B*) Coronal CT scan in patient postprocedure. (*C, D*) This technique allows for binostril ([*C*] through left nostril and [*D*] through right nostril) bimanual instrumentation. Dotted line in (*A*) depicts location of the superior septectomy. *Red arrow* in (*A*) depicts limited lateral reach through the ipsilateral left nostril. *Blue arrow* in (*A*) depicts improvement in lateral reach through the contralateral nostril by using the superior septectomy window. (© 2015 Chris Gralapp, Fairfax, CA.)

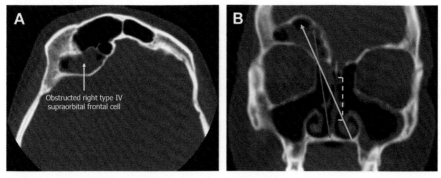

Fig. 3. (*A*) Axial and (*B*) coronal CT scans of a patient with an obstructed right frontal sinus. There is improved access with Eloy IIC (*green arrow*), with white bracket showing the septectomy window, compared with standard ipsilateral approach (*red arrow*). (© 2013 American Academy of Otolaryngology – Head and Neck Surgery Foundation, Alexandria, VA; with permission.)

binostril and bimanual dissection is of particular importance in cases of soft tissue tumors of the lateral frontal sinus recess or surpraorbital ethmoid.

Modified Mini-Lothrop Procedure (Eloy IID)

The modified mini-Lothrop procedure (Eloy IID) is a procedure intended to treat frontal sinus disease when ipsilateral access to the frontal sinus recess is not possible.[9,10] Ipsilateral access to the frontal sinus recess can be hindered by one of many circumstances, including scarring, outflow tract osteogenesis, or fat prolapse from previous medial orbital wall decompression or trauma (**Fig. 4**). The procedure combines the removal of the contralateral frontal sinus floor (Draf IIB) and an endoscopic frontal intersinus septectomy (**Fig. 5**). Although the modified Lothrop procedure, as originally described, did not require a complete intersinus septectomy, it is desirable to perform a total intersinus septectomy in the modified mini-Lothrop procedure (Eloy IID) because this window is designed to be the contralateral diseased frontal sinus' only drainage pathway.

Modified Subtotal-Lothrop Procedure (Eloy IIE)

The modified subtotal-Lothrop procedure (Eloy IIE) is designed for the treatment of recalcitrant bilateral frontal sinus disease and ipsilateral anterior skull base lesion resection, with an emphasis on preserving as much of the normal sinonasal architecture as possible (**Fig. 6**).[11,12] This procedure can be used for large posterior frontal

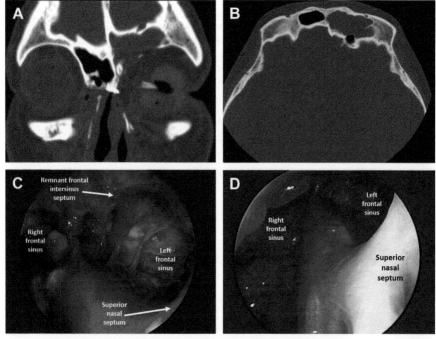

Fig. 4. (*A*) Coronal and (*B*) axial CT scans in a patient with orbital fat prolapse. (*C*) Intraoperative view of nasal cavity and sinus immediately after Eloy IID or modified mini-Lothrop procedure. (*D*) Eight-month postoperative nasal endoscopic view of the sinonasal cavity after the Eloy IID procedure. (© 2012 American Rhinological Society – American Academy of Otolaryngic Allergy, Reston, VA; with permission.)

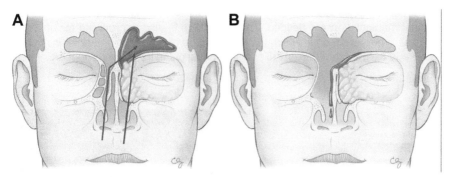

Fig. 5. (*A*) Artwork in the coronal-plane demonstrating Eloy IID (*blue arrow*) in a patient with fat prolapse preventing an ipsilateral frontal sinusotomy (*red arrow*). (*B*) Depiction of drainage via the contralateral nasal cavity after the Eloy IID procedure. (© 2011 Chris Gralapp, Fairfax, CA.)

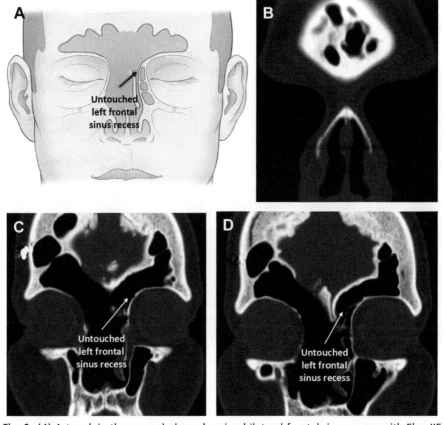

Fig. 6. (*A*) Artwork in the coronal plane showing bilateral frontal sinus access with Eloy IIE (modified subtotal-Lothrop procedure) with preservation of the contralateral frontal sinus recess. (*B–D*) Coronal CT scans of patient postoperatively after tumor resection using Eloy IIE. (*B*) Intact anterior septum, (*C*) access to both frontal sinuses, and (*D*) intact contralateral frontal sinus recess are seen. (© 2014 Chris Gralapp, Fairfax, CA.)

sinus encephaloceles in which access to the bilateral posterior frontal sinus table and bimanual manipulation are desired. This technique is also appropriate for unilateral sinonasal tumor resection in which the contralateral frontal sinus recess is uninvolved (**Figs. 7** and **8**). The procedure involves the removal of the frontal sinus floor unilaterally

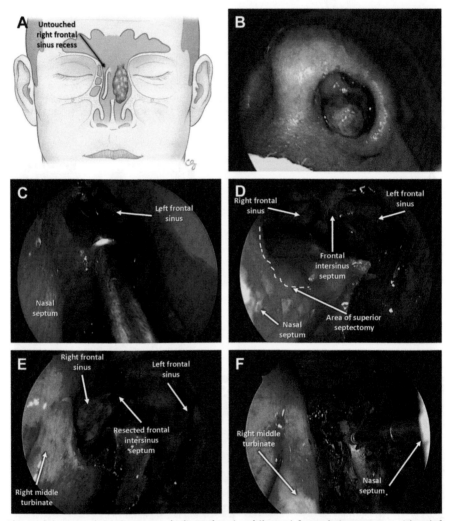

Fig. 7. (*A*) Artwork in the coronal plane showing bilateral frontal sinus access with a left Eloy IIE (modified subtotal-Lothrop procedure) with preservation of contralateral frontal recess. Endonasal view of intraoperative modified subtotal-Lothrop procedure in a patient with an olfactory neuroblastoma, (*B*) Initial intraoperative view of the lesion. (*C*) Using a 30° rigid endoscope, a left Draf IIB is performed. (*D*) A superior septectomy is performed and the medial contralateral frontal sinus floor is resected. (*E*) The intersinus septectomy is subsequently performed. The right (contralateral) frontal sinus recess as well as the right middle turbinate are preserved. (*F*) View from the contralateral (*right*) nasal cavity after completion of left Draf IIB, superior septectomy, and intersinus septectomy. (© 2014 American Rhinological Society – American Academy of Otolaryngic Allergy, Reston, VA; with permission.)

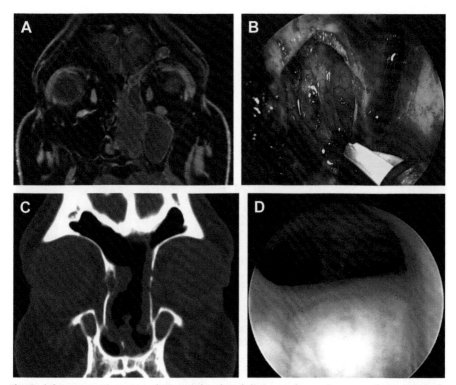

Fig. 8. (*A*) Preoperative coronal T1-weighted gadolinium enhanced paranasal sinus MRI of a patient with a left sinonasal olfactory neuroblastoma. (*B*) Intraoperative endoscopic view of the anterior skull base defect after tumor resection. (*C*) Coronal postoperative CT scan of the same patient showing a patent modified subtotal-Lothrop procedure (Eloy IIE). (*D*) Six-month postoperative endoscopic image of the patent frontal sinus cavity. (© 2014 American Rhinological Society – American Academy of Otolaryngic Allergy, Reston, VA; with permission.)

(Draf IIB) with the addition of a superior septectomy and an intersinus septectomy. This allows for access and visualization of the ipsilateral and contralateral frontal sinus and binostril and bimanual instrumentation (Video 1). The contralateral frontal sinus recess and contralateral middle turbinate are left undisturbed.

Modified Central-Lothrop Procedure (Eloy IIF)

The modified central-Lothrop procedure (Eloy IIF) has not been previously described in the literature. In this procedure, emphasis is on preserving as much of the normal sinonasal architecture as feasible (**Figs. 9** and **10**). The procedure involves the removal of the medial frontal sinus floor bilaterally with the addition of a superior septectomy and an intersinus septectomy. This allows for access and visualization of both frontal sinuses and affords binostril and bimanual instrumentation. This procedure can be

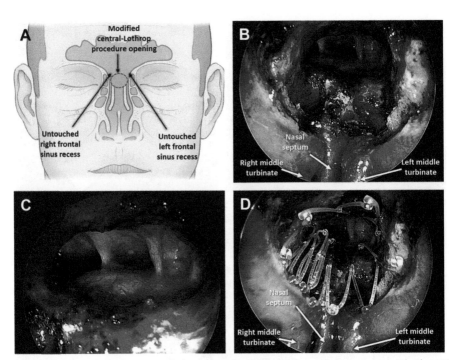

Fig. 9. (*A*) Artwork in the coronal plane showing bilateral frontal sinus access with Eloy IIF (modified central-Lothrop procedure) with preservation of the bilateral frontal sinus recesses. (*B*) Intraoperative 30° endoscopic view of the modified central-Lothrop procedure (Eloy IIF). (*C*) Close-up view of the central opening. (*D*) Endoscopic view of steroid eluting stent placement. (© 2015 Chris Gralapp, Fairfax, CA.)

used for frontal sinus disease located near the midline. It can result in scarring and subsequent obstruction of the created central opening. However, preservation of both frontal sinus recesses lateral to the midline opening, and resection of the frontal intersinus septum should allow ample communication between the two sides with an exit pathway in either of the untouched frontal sinus recess.

SUMMARY

Current classification of endonasal frontal sinus drainage and access techniques include the Draf and nasofrontal approaches. These classification systems do not include 3 recently published modifications (modified hemi-Lothrop procedure, modified mini-Lothrop procedure, and modified subtotal-Lothrop procedure) and the currently described additional modification (modified central-Lothrop procedure). For this reason, a new classification system has been proposed, which consolidates the 2 previous methods and includes the 4 new techniques.

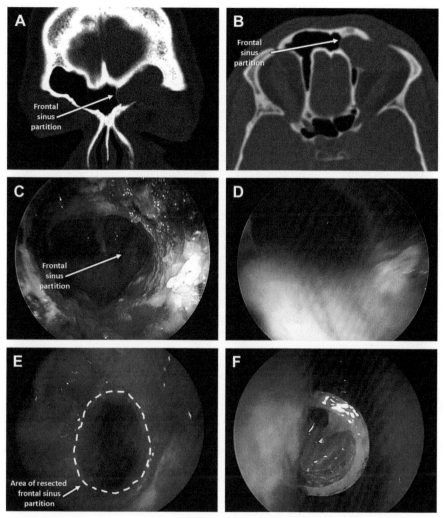

Fig. 10. Preoperative (*A*) coronal and (*B*) axial CT scans of a patient with proptosis and a right fronto-orbital mucopyocele causing destruction of the superomedial orbital wall. Note the partition separating the mucopyocele and the frontal sinus. This lesion was approached via a modified central-Lothrop procedure (Eloy IIF). (*C*) Intraoperative endoscopic view of the modified central-Lothrop procedure (Eloy IIF) prior to the resection of the dividing partition. (*D*) Copious mucopurulent extravasation is noted after resection of the partition. (*E*) Depiction of the opening after resection of the partition. (*F*) A sialastic splint is used to stent the created opening after adequate drainage of the mucopyocele.

SUPPLEMENTARY DATA

Supplementary data related to this article can be found at http://dx.doi.org/10.1016/j. otc.2016.03.023.

REFERENCES

1. Javer AR, Alandejani T. Prevention and management of complications in frontal sinus surgery. Otolaryngol Clin North Am 2010;43:827–38.

2. Draf W. Endonasal micro-endoscopic frontal sinus surgery: the fulda concept. Operat Tech Otolaryngol Head Neck Surg 1991;2:234–40.
3. Gross WE, Gross CW, Becker D, et al. Modified transnasal endoscopic Lothrop procedure as an alternative to frontal sinus obliteration. Otolaryngol Head Neck Surg 1995;113:427–34.
4. Close LG, Lee NK, Leach JL, et al. Endoscopic resection of the intranasal frontal sinus floor. Ann Otol Rhinol Laryngol 1994;103:952–8.
5. Eloy JA, Friedel ME, Murray KP, et al. Modified hemi-Lothrop procedure for supra-orbital frontal sinus access: a cadaveric feasibility study. Otolaryngol Head Neck Surg 2011;145:489–93.
6. Eloy JA, Kuperan AB, Friedel ME, et al. Modified hemi-lothrop procedure for su-praorbital frontal sinus access: a case series. Otolaryngol Head Neck Surg 2012; 147:167–9.
7. Friedel ME, Li S, Langer PD, et al. Modified hemi-lothrop procedure for supraor-bital ethmoid lesion access. Laryngoscope 2012;122:442–4.
8. Liu JK, Mendelson ZS, Dubal PM, et al. The modified hemi-Lothrop procedure: a variation of the endoscopic endonasal approach for resection of a supraorbital psammomatoid ossifying fibroma. J Clin Neurosci 2014;21:2233–8.
9. Eloy JA, Friedel ME, Kuperan AB, et al. Modified mini-lothrop/extended draf IIb procedure for contralateral frontal sinus disease: a cadaveric feasibility study. Otolaryngol Head Neck Surg 2012;146:165–8.
10. Eloy JA, Friedel ME, Kuperan AB, et al. Modified mini-lothrop/extended draf IIB procedure for contralateral frontal sinus disease: a case series. Int Forum Allergy Rhinol 2012;2:321–4.
11. Eloy JA, Liu JK, Choudhry OJ, et al. Modified subtotal lothrop procedure for extended frontal sinus and anterior skull base access: a cadaveric feasibility study with clinical correlates. J Neurol Surg B Skull Base 2013;74:130–5.
12. Eloy JA, Mady LJ, Kanumuri VV, et al. Modified subtotal-Lothrop procedure for extended frontal sinus and anterior skull-base access: a case series. Int Forum Allergy Rhinol 2014;4:517–22.
13. Weber R, Draf W, Kratzsch B, et al. Modern concepts of frontal sinus surgery. Laryngoscope 2001;111:137–46.

Outcomes After Frontal Sinus Surgery

An Evidence-Based Review

Adam S. DeConde, MD[a], Timothy L. Smith, MD, MPH[b],*

KEYWORDS

- Draf IIa • Draf III • Endoscopic frontal sinusotomy • Endoscopic modified Lothrop
- Frontal sinusitis • Frontal sinus obliteration • Endoscopic sinus surgery
- Frontal sinus drillout

KEY POINTS

- Frontal sinusotomy via Draf IIa is effective for most patients with medically refractory frontal sinusitis based on reported case series.
- Endoscopic postoperative patency rates of Draf IIa surgery is significantly higher in patients who intraoperatively achieved diameter no smaller than 4.5 mm.
- Frontal sinus closure by either cicatricial stenosis or polypoid edema is associated with persistent symptoms after Draf IIa.
- Draf III is an effective salvage operation for patients that avoids some of the morbidities associated with frontal sinus obliteration.
- Short-term (2-year) neo-ostial patency rates are high and are associated with high rates of symptom control.

INTRODUCTION

Chronic rhinosinusitis (CRS) is a common disease that carries significant impairment of patient quality of life (QOL)[1] and patient productivity.[2] CRS can frequently be treated successfully with medical therapy, but patients that have persistent bothersome

Potential Conflicts of Interest: None to report.

Financial Disclosures: T.L. Smith is supported by a grant for this investigation from the National Institute on Deafness and Other Communication Disorders, one of the National Institutes of Health, Bethesda, Maryland (R01 DC005805; PI/PD: T.L. Smith). T.L. Smith and A.S. DeConde are consultants for IntersectENT (Menlo Park, CA), which is not affiliated with or discussed in this article.

[a] Division of Otolaryngology-Head and Neck Surgery, Department of Surgery, University of California-San Diego, 200 W Arbor Dr., MC 8895, San Diego, CA 92103-8895, USA; [b] Division of Rhinology, Sinus, and Skull Base Surgery, Department of Otolaryngology-Head and Neck Surgery, Oregon Sinus Center, Oregon Health & Science University, 3181 Southwest Sam Jackson Park Road, PV-01, Portland, OR 97239, USA

* Corresponding author.

E-mail address: smithtim@ohsu.edu

Otolaryngol Clin N Am 49 (2016) 1019–1033

http://dx.doi.org/10.1016/j.otc.2016.03.024

oto.theclinics.com

symptoms despite maximal medical therapy can elect to undergo surgical treatment of the sinuses. The primary goal of endoscopic sinus surgery (ESS) is to provide improvement in the QOL of patients that have failed medical therapy.[3,4]

ESS is thought to deliver improvements in QOL through improved control of the underlying inflammatory process. Since its inception, ESS has been predicated on creation of durable openings into the sinuses that allow for efficient drainage of sinus secretions.[5] Understanding of the underlying pathophysiology of CRS has broadened, and a secondary goal of sinus surgery is control of the intrinsic mucosal inflammation of the sinuses through delivery of topical therapies.[6] Patent sinusotomies, therefore, are thought to be a critical goal in control of the underlying inflammatory process.

Surgical interventions of the frontal sinus offer a unique surgical challenge because of the idiosyncrasies of the frontal sinus outflow tract anatomy. The frontal sinuses rest above the frontal beak in the frontal bone with an outflow tract nestled between the orbits laterally and skull base medially. These fundamental limits of dissection provide what are frequently the most narrow sinusotomy and the highest risk for major complications and stenosis. Historical approaches to the frontal sinuses, including the Lynch and Lothrop procedures, had high short-term patency rates, but over time developed 30% failure rates in the long-term.[7] These failure rates elevated the osteoplastic flap with frontal sinus obliteration to the putative gold standard[7]; however, the osteoplastic flap is associated with significant morbidity including supraorbital neuralgia, frontal bossing, abdominal fat donor site complications, and difficulty with surveillance of the sinus.[8]

With the advent of ESS reasonable surgical alternatives to the open approaches were developed. Draf[9] described a range of potential interventions from merely performing a total ethmoidectomy without any intervention on the frontal recess (Draf I), to complete clearing of the frontal recess (Draf IIA), and finally an extended sinusotomy that marsupializes the bilateral frontal sinuses through a transeptal removal of the frontal sinus floors and intersinus septum (Draf III) (**Table 1**). A variety of modifications of these techniques exist, but the critical difference between the various techniques is whether the sinusotomy can be performed with hand instrumentation or requires a drill. Use of a drill requires stripped mucosa, which has been associated with high rates of restenosis[7] and higher rates of complications on prior surgeries. Therefore, for the purposes of this article, these two types of endoscopic frontal sinus surgery are evaluated separately.

This article summarizes the evidence underpinning surgical intervention of the frontal sinus. Special attention is given to the impact of frontal sinus surgery on

Table 1	
Description and terminology of frontal sinusotomies	
Frontal Sinusotomies	**Description**
Draf I	Total ethmoidectomy with no instrumentation of the narrowest part of the frontal recess
Draf IIa	Mucosal-sparing clearance of the frontal recess of tissue
Draf IIb	Removal of the superior anterior attachment of the head of the middle to the septum turbinate and the floor of the frontal sinus
Extended Draf IIB/unilateral drillout	A Draf IIb that includes unilateral drilling away of the frontal beak
Draf III	Removal of the frontal intersinus septum, the frontal beak, and the superior septum

patient-centered QOL measures, and the effectiveness of surgical interventions at creating a lasting patent frontal sinusotomy as measured by either endosocopic or radiographic data.

EVIDENCE SUPPORTING USE OF ENDOSCOPIC SINUS SURGERY FOR CHRONIC RHINOSINUSITIS

In determining the efficacy or effectiveness of an intervention one should consider how that intervention does relative to a comparison group. In the case of frontal sinusotomy, and ESS in general, one could consider that medical therapy is a reasonable comparison. With this in mind, before an investigation of the evidence underlying frontal sinusotomy, a quick review of the evidence supporting ESS over continued medical therapy is warranted.

A randomized controlled trial of medical therapy versus ESS might ideally compare outcomes and differences between these two interventions but several important barriers exist to executing such a trial. Patients being considered for ESS have failed medical therapy, and randomizing patients to an already failed therapy would likely impair enrollment. Furthermore, one could argue that such an issue is past clinical equipoise given that multi-institutional prospective cohort studies have demonstrated that patients that have failed medical therapy improve after ESS.[10–12]

It has only been in the last handful of years that comparative effectiveness studies comparing ESS with medical therapy have begun to emerge.[13–15] Comparative effectiveness studies are a more pragmatic real-world approach to comparing two interventions that are observational in nature. Selection treatment bias exists because there is no randomization protocol, but this is the reality of the application of medicine and therefore offers greater external validity. The early comparative effectiveness data do support that patients with medically recalcitrant CRS are approximately three times more likely (odds ratio, 3.37; 95% confidence interval, 1.27–8.90; $P = .014$) to experience improvement on disease-specific validated QOL outcome measures.[13] Patients electing surgical therapy are more likely to resolve thick nasal discharge, nasal obstruction, and facial pain/pressure than patients pursuing only continued medical therapy,[14] but no difference for olfaction outcomes.[15]

Given the growing body of literature favoring ESS over continued medical management in patients with medically refractory CRS, perhaps, ideally, a study designed to determine the efficacy of frontal sinusotomy would randomize patients to ESS with or without frontal sinusotomy. Problems exist with this methodology as well, in that it could be fairly argued that it is unethical to randomize patients with frontal sinus disease present on preoperative imaging or intraoperative endoscopy away from frontal sinusotomy based on prior retrospective case series showing that persistent frontal sinus disease can lead to persistent symptoms.[16] There may just be such a large effect size associated with addressing the other sinuses on QOL measures, that the differential impact of presence or absence of a frontal sinusotomy could be obfuscated on a QOL questionnaire.[17] Endoscopic data may be the key to determining the difference in the outcomes, but this is admittedly not a patient-centered outcome measure because this was found to be different in patients undergoing surgery with and without frontal sinusotomy.[17]

With these limitations in mind, the following review of the evidence underlying frontal sinusotomy is placed into adequate context. The evidence level consists entirely of single institution retrospective case series. The outcomes include subjective measures of QOL of a variety of qualities and frequency of patency of the frontal sinusotomy at follow-up on either endoscopy or imaging.

Key Points

- Level 2 evidence supports use of ESS for patients with CRS with inadequately controlled symptoms on maximal medical therapy.
- Understanding the impact of the extent of ESS with or without frontal sinusotomy on QOL measures is challenging to capture because of the large effect size of any surgical intervention.

EVIDENCE SUPPORTING USE OF DRAF IIa FRONTAL SINUSOTOMY

All of the data examining the outcomes of frontal sinusotomy (specifically, Draf IIa) are level IV evidence (**Table 2**).[16,18–31] A wide range of methodologies was used to capture subjective and objective outcomes. Unfortunately, validated disease-specific measures were rarely used even in the later studies by which time such instruments were widely available. Patency rates for the most part were determined by postoperative nasal endoscopy with visualization of some portion of the frontal sinus cavity as the requirement for a patent sinusotomy. Furthermore, comparison across these studies is impaired by a lack of consistent reporting of patient baseline characteristics.

Given these caveats, most patients undergoing frontal sinusotomies in the literature report symptomatic improvement (68.5%–92%). Patency rates of frontal sinusotomy ranged widely (27.3%–92%), but within the last 10 years the range narrowed to 67.6% to 92% with most studies reporting endoscopic patency in the mid-80% endoscopic success rates.

These studies span 25 years of investigation of the topic, which is remarkable considering how much technology and technique have evolved over that time. Since the first study was performed, a variety of new technologies have become near ubiquitous. The first study describing use of the microdebrider emerged in 1997.[22] Other innovations that are not always explicitly mentioned in the studies but have permeated the specialty during this timeline include mucosal-sparing technique, introduction of image guidance, topical steroid irrigations, drug-eluting stents, and high-definition cameras. The clinical significance of any one of these interventions is not always clear, but some permutation of each of these innovations likely exists in a modern day surgical armamentarium. It is encouraging to see a general trend in improvement in outcomes between the studies from the 1990s and from the 2000s and 2010s. It does seem that the endoscopic patency rate postoperatively is more reliable with 67.6% to 92% reported in the last 10 years in contrast to the first 10 years, which ranges from 27.3% to 100% (see **Table 2**).

Patency rates for the most part were determined by postoperative nasal endoscopy with angled scopes with direct visualization into the cavity for the most part as a binary outcome. Postoperative frontal sinus outflow tracts, however, can obstruct with either swelling of soft tissue and/or polyp recurrence or through cicatricial scar formation. This may be an important distinction, because it could be argued that sinuses failing from cicatricial scar may be secondary to technique and may benefit from an intervention, such as refined surgical technique and/or possible stenting, whereas polyp recurrence may result from failure to control intrinsic mucosal disease, which might improve with control of mucosal inflammation and may benefit from refinement of topical therapies. Future study would ideally clarify how stenosis occurs to better guide interventions.

There may also be some threshold of sinusotomy dimensions that are sufficient to maintain an open sinus, and Chandra and colleagues[28] postulate that a diameter of 4 to 5 mm results in a sinus that is likely to maintain patency. Naidoo and colleagues[16] examined the size of endoscopic sinusotomy and found statistically significant difference in mean smallest dimension of the frontal sinusotomy in patients that went on to stenose and those that remained patent (95% confidence interval, 2.94–4.47 and 4.60–5.15, respectively; $P = .0068$). The only difference identified was in the size of frontal sinusotomy and based on the confidence intervals the likelihood of closure of a sinusotomy greater than 4.5 mm is quite unlikely.

There does seem to be a threshold of sinusotomy size beyond which the likelihood of closure drops significantly. Hosemann and colleagues[23] found that when the diameter of the ostium dropped below 5 mm the stenosis rate increased from 16% to 30%. Stenosis rates rapidly increased as the diameter dropped with sinuses with 2-mm diameters resulting in stenosis in 50% of the sinusotomies. When comparing the intraoperative and postoperative diameters, a mean decrease of 1.1 mm was observed (from 5.6 mm to 3.5 mm), representing a relative reduction of 37.5% of the diameter. Preoperative imaging often can clue the surgeon into the fundamental limits of a frontal recess dissection and inherently narrowed anatomy may be one variable that can preoperatively forecast failure.

Maximization of the frontal sinusotomy is a critical goal of surgical intervention, but this opening must not come at the expense of mucosal preservation. This dogma is not based on a large evidence base, but early experience with mucosal trauma via external approaches led to high frontal sinus failure rates.[7] The findings are reiterated in some of the early Draf IIa surgeries before the complete evolution of modern surgical endoscopic technique. Wigand and Hosemann[19] reported high rates of frontal sinus stenosis (40%), but report using a drill in approximately 50% of the cases. There was a relatively low threshold to use a diamond drill in unilateral procedures to maximize the outflow tract, which may explain the high rate of stenosis. The impact of mucosal trauma may be reflected in increasing stenosis rates of the small-diameter frontal sinusotomies. As sinusotomies approach the diameters of instrumentation the risk of iatrogenic mucosal trauma increases. Careful technique and appropriate instrumentation may decrease the risk of cicatricial stenosis.

Although the size of the frontal sinusotomy likely plays an important role in patent frontal sinuses, it is conceivable that the underlying inflammatory process also influences success and failure. Remarkably, there was no difference between patients with patent and stenosed frontal sinusotomies in rates of nasal polyposis, eosinophilic mucin, asthma, Lund-Mackay Score (overall and frontal sinus-specific), and prevalence in allergy in the study by Naidoo and colleagues.[16] Askar and colleagues[31] did no statistical analysis of the subtypes of disease, but the patency rate seems comparable across the board regardless of statistical significance with 88.4% of patients with CRS with nasal polyps, 91.9% of patients with CRS without nasal polyps, 88.9% of patients with allergic fungal sinusitis, and 100% of mucoceles remaining patient. These data are somewhat surprising because there has really been such an emphasis on the importance of controlling intrinsic mucosal inflammation with topical steroids,[6] and there is optimism that control of dysbiosis may prevent sinusitis recurrence and/or persistence.[32] One could speculate that perhaps the effect size of a large sinusotomy washes out the impact of the severity of the mucosal inflammation. Or perhaps the studies have not identified the best variables to measure intrinsic mucosal inflammation or scar formation. No data exist on the impact of the tissue eosinophilia or osteoneogenesis on frontal sinusotomy stenosis, both of which have been linked together and to diminished postoperative gains in QOL.[33,34] Larger sample sizes that could power the detection of differences on multivariate analysis patient characteristics on endoscopic outcomes would be required to clarify this issue.

Understanding the impact of frontal sinusotomy on subjective outcomes is challenging to capture and isolate because so frequently frontal sinusotomy is combined

Table 2
Evidence summary of Draf IIa frontal sinusotomy

Study, Year	Study Design	LOE	Number of Subjects	Procedures	Mean Follow-up (mo)	Objective Outcome	Objective Outcome Success Rate	Subjective Outcome	Subjective Outcome Success Rate
Schaefer & Close,[18] 1990	RCS	IV	36	Frontal sinusotomy	16.4	Endoscopy and/or CT	21/36 patent	Nonvalidated measures	21/36 resolved, 11/36 improved
Wigand & Hosemann,[19] 1991	RCS	IV	220	126 sinus drillouts	41	Endoscopic patency	40%	NA	NA
Moriyama et al,[20] 1994	RCS	IV	57	Frontal sinusotomy	6–41 (range)	Endoscopic patency	73.40%	NA	NA
Christmas & Krouse,[21] 1996	RCS	IV	30	Frontal sinusotomy	NA	Endoscopic patency	100%	NA	NA
Jacobs,[22] 1997	RCS	IV	101	Frontal sinusotomy	16	Endoscopic patency	27.3% of patients with polyps, 76.9% without polyps	Nonvalidated	85% reported improvement
Hosemann et al,[23] 1997	RCS	IV	110	Frontal sinusotomy	13	Endoscopic probing	81%	Nonvalidated	87% report improvement
Metson & Glicklich,[24] 1998	PCS	IV	63	24 frontal drillouts	22.7	Need for revision surgery	87.5% did not require obliteration	CSS and SF-36	Statistically significant improvement in CSS and SF-36

Study	Design	LOE	N	Procedure	Follow-up	Objective Outcome	Value	Subjective Measure	Value
Wormald,[25] 2002	PCS	IV	64	Frontal sinusotomy	15.4	Endoscopic patency	82%	Nonvalidated measures	82% resolved symptoms
Wormald & Chan,[26] 2003	RCS	IV	44 (13 Draf IIIs)	13 Draf IIIs	12	Endoscopic patency	100%	Nonvalidated measures	82% resolved symptoms
Chiu & Vaughan,[27] 2004	RCS	IV	67	Frontal sinusotomy	32	Endoscopic patency	86.60%	RSOM-31	Mean improvement of 57% on RSOM-31 (30% = clinically meaningful)
Chandra et al,[28] 2004	RCS	IV	66	Frontal sinusotomy	8.3	Endoscopic patency	82.30%	Nonvalidated measures	NA
Friedman et al,[29] 2006	RCS	IV	157	Frontal sinusotomy	72.3	Endoscopic patency	67.60%	Nonvalidated measures	92% improved
Chan et al,[30] 2009	RCS	IV	161	Frontal sinusotomy	45.9	Endoscopic patency	88%	SNOT-20	68.5% improved
Naidoo et al,[16] 2012	RCS	IV	109	Frontal sinusotomy	16.2	Endoscopic patency	92%	Nonvalidated measures	85/109 resolved, 78%
Askar et al,[31] 2015	PCS	IV	60	Frontal sinusotomy	10	Endoscopic patency	90%	RSDI	—

Abbreviations: CSS, chronic sinusitis survey; CT, computed tomography; LOE, level of evidence; NA, not available; PCS, prospective case series; RCS, retrospective case series; RSDI, rhinosinusitis disability index; RSOM-31, Rhinosinusitis Outcome Measures; SF-36, Short Form-36; SNOT, sinonasal outcome test.
Data from Refs.[16,18–31]

in conjunction with other surgical interventions. Achieving a clinically meaningful difference on a disease-specific outcome measure is a higher bar to clear and a prospective cohort analysis did not find that the extent of surgery achieved clinical significance.[17] A comparison of patients that had frontal sinusotomies that stenosed found they were more likely to have persistent sinonasal symptoms.[16] An examination of patients electing revision sinus surgery demonstrated that retained cells narrowing the frontal recess and/or middle turbinate lateralization was present in most patients.[35] Although the data on the subjective outcomes of frontal sinusotomy of CRS cannot demonstrate efficacy, there is concern that failure to completely address the sinuses may lead to increased stenosis, increased symptoms, and potentially revision surgery.

Although the level of evidence remains low, and the volume of patients studied remains low, there are some critical learning points from the frontal sinusotomy Draf IIa literature. Maximization of the frontal sinusotomy is critical to prevent stenosis, and really one of the few variables in the control of the surgeon. This opening should ideally be greater than 4.5 mm, because such a sinusotomy is unlikely to stenose regardless of the underlying pathology. Subjects with inherently narrow outflow tracts that cannot be augmented to such a size secondary to close orbits and/or close frontal beak are at high risk of failure with a Draf IIa technique. These patients are recognized preoperatively on imaging, and should be counseled that they are at increased risk for possibly needing an extended sinusotomy as a salvage operation. Furthermore, the optimization of the frontal sinusotomy diameter should not come at the cost of mucosal stripping because this can predispose to cicatricial scarring. Appropriately and surgically successfully addressing the frontal sinus may decrease postoperative symptom burden because frontal sinusotomy stenosis is associated with persistent symptoms. Retained frontal sinus cells have also been reported at high rates seeking revision surgery.

The decision to perform a frontal sinusotomy is likely different in the hands of each surgeon because the risk-benefit analysis of potential gains must be weighed against each surgeon's comfort level with frontal sinusotomy. Induction of iatrogenic cicatricial scarring, or worse, orbital or neurologic complications, is a risk that is unique to each surgeon and as a profession currently relies on each individual surgeon to judge what intervention optimizes patient outcomes.

Key Points

- The level of evidence for the effectiveness of Draf IIa frontal sinusotomy is entirely composed of case series.
- The available evidence demonstrates that Draf IIa mucosal-sparing openings greater than 4.5 mm in diameter have a very high patency rate postoperatively.
- Stenosis of the frontal sinus is associated with persistent symptoms.

EVIDENCE SUPPORTING USE OF DRAF III FRONTAL SINUSOTOMY

Although the Draf IIa has shown high rates of patency, a variety of situations may arise that might make a Draf IIa not feasible or eventually fail. Therefore, a clear understanding of the optimal salvage surgery is critical to any surgeon embarking on surgical treatment of the frontal sinus. An open approach to the frontal sinus with removal of the frontal bone was first described by Reidel in 1889, and modified in the 1950s with preservation of the osteoplastic flap and stripping of the sinus mucosa with subsequent obliteration of the sinus.[36] The goal of frontal sinus obliteration is to achieve a scarred and nonfunctional sinus while preserving cosmesis and achieves such a success in 75% to 93% of patients.[37] Frontal sinus obliteration, however, is not without morbidity. The procedure takes longer and has higher blood loss than the Draf III,[37] and late mucocele formation is detected on MRI in 10% of patients.[38] Other late complications include numbness of V1 (8.5%), frontal embossment (3.4%), insufficient esthetic results (5.1%), extrusion of allograft obliteration material (3.4%), and depression of the frontal table (6.8%).[38]

The Draf III seeks to provide a less morbid approach with comparable efficacy. Draf described the procedure in 1991[9] and its application was reported in 1995 by Gross and colleagues[39] as an alternative to frontal sinus obliteration. The modern day Draf III is a modification of Draf's description of removing the superior septum and frontal intersinus septum along with all frontal recess cells. Removal of the frontal beak with a drill provides a much larger opening to the frontal sinus, but does come at the trade-off of mucosal stripping. The true fundamental limits of the Draf III are from the first olfactory fiber posteriorly and the periosteum laterally and anteriorly.[40]

The literature on Draf III frontal sinusotomies is similar to that on the Draf IIa consisting predominantly of case series from single institutions (**Table 3**)[8,24,26,39,41–60] with similar outcomes. In some ways, however, more evidence has been published on this salvage surgery that is required in only a minority of patients with CRS. A systematic review on the safety and efficacy of the Draf III found that endoscopic patency rates were high (95.9% of 354 available for endoscopic evaluation) at 28.5 months postoperatively.[61] Similarly, improvement in symptoms was achieved in 82.2% of patients. These are impressive results for a salvage operation. However, long-term data show that the neo-ostium decreases in size for up to 2 years after surgery,[59,60] which requires at least as long of a follow-up to draw conclusions about patency outcomes. There is a trend in longer follow-up for the endoscopic patency rates in the recent literature, which are critical data given the need to leave exposed bone when drilling out the frontal beak. Therefore, the discussion of this review is focused on truly long-term data, defined by greater than 2-year follow-up, because the long-term results of the Draf III is where the controversy remains.

Two recent studies examining the long-term endoscopic outcomes vary widely in patency rates. Naidoo and colleagues[59] reported on 229 patients that underwent Draf III procedures with mean follow-up of 45 months. Endoscopic patency rates of the neo-ostium occurred in 221 out of 229 (97%) patients. Measurements of the neo-ostial axes found mean dimensions of 21.0 mm × 19.5 mm. Neo-ostia stabilized after 2 years. Ting and colleagues[60] report another long-term study examining outcomes of 143 patients with a mean follow-up of 10.2 years. Although the retrospective nature of this study precluded endoscopic measurement of neo-ostia over time, the end point need for revision surgery found that 29.9% of patients went on to require revision surgery. Although the Ting study does report on a longer timeline, most of these revisions occurred within the first 5 years. This experience is in stark contrast to the 5.2% revision surgery rate reported by Naidoo and colleagues.[59] The experience of Ting and colleagues[60] is more in line with the prior study with Casiano and Livinston[42] reporting 43% stenosing by more than 50% within 6 months of surgery. Tran and colleagues[53] also reported a mean stenosis of 33% of the neo-ostium cross-sectional area that continued out to 1 year.

Subjective outcomes mirror the objective findings. The long-term data reported by Naidoo and colleagues[59] used a validated sinus-specific subjective measure that found 47% of patients were asymptomatic postoperatively and another 27% reported only mild symptoms. A minority of subjects had severe symptoms (8%), but there was no worsening of symptoms after Draf III. These data are again in stark contrast to the high rate of patients electing revision surgery in the Ting study.

Naidoo and colleagues[59] offer some theories as to the success of their Draf IIIs. The large neo-ostium achieved may allow for increased delivery of topical therapies and

Table 3
Evidence summary of Draf III frontal sinusotomy

Study, Year	Study Design	LOE	N	Study Groups	Mean Follow-up (mo)	Revision Surgery, N (%)
Gross et al,[39] 1995	RCS	IV	10	Draf III	7	0 (0)
Gross et al,[41] 1997	Comparative OPF cohort	III	20	OPF, Draf III	12	0 (0)
Casiano & Livingston,[42] 1998	RCS	IV	21	Draf III	NA	2 (9.5)
Metson & Gliklich,[24] 1998	RCS	IV	9	Draf III	22.7	0 (0)
Kikawada et al,[43] 1999	RCS	IV	16	Draf III	23.3	2 (13)[a]
McLaughlin et al,[44] 1999	RCS	IV	20	Draf III	12	0 (0)
Ulualp et al,[45] 2000	Comparative OPF cohort	III	15	OPF, Draf III	6–30 (range)	2 (13)
Schulze et al,[46] 2002	RCS	IV	13	Draf III	34.5	2 (15)
Schlosser et al,[47] 2002	RCS	IV	54	Draf III	40.3	17 (32)
Samaha et al,[48] 2003	RCS	IV	66	Draf III	49.2	10 (15)
Stankiewicz & Wachter,[49] 2003	RCS	IV	10	Draf III	34	5 (50)
Wormald et al,[50] 2003	RCS	IV	16	Draf III	18.9	1 (6.3)
Wormald & Chan,[26] 2003	RCS	IV	13	Draf III	NA	0 (0)

Wormald,[8] 2003	RCS	IV	83	Draf III	21.9	6 (7.2)
Khong et al,[51] 2004	RCS	IV	21	Draf III	NA	2 (9.5)
Banhiran et al,[52] 2006	RCS	IV	72	Draf III	22	5 (6.9)
Tran et al,[53] 2007	RCS	IV	77	Draf III	29.2	10 (13)
Shirazi et al,[54] 2007	RCS	IV	97	Draf III	18	22 (23)
Nakagawa & Ito,[55] 2007	RCS	IV	6	Draf III	24.5	0 (0)
Eloy et al,[56] 2011	RCS	IV	120	Draf III	24.6	15 (13)[a]
Georgalas et al,[57] 2011	RCS	IV	122	Draf III	NA	39 (32)
Hildenbrand et al,[58] 2012	RCS	IV	24	Draf III	25.6	1 (4.2)
Naidoo et al,[59] 2014	RCS	IV	229	Draf III	45	12 (5.2)
Ting et al,[60] 2014	RCS	IV	204	Extended Draf IIb (n = 61), and Draf III (n = 143)	120	61 (30)

Abbreviations: LOE, level of evidence; NA, not available; OPF, osteoplastic flap; RCS, retrospective case series.
[a] End point reported is endoscopic closure, not revision surgery.
Data from Refs. 8,24,26,39,41–60

increase the volume of irrigation preventing accumulation of discharge. The large neo-ostium's reported by Naidoo and colleagues may also allow for greater cicatricial scarring or tissue edema without leading to a complete stenosis. An examination of the mean neo-ostium created intraoperatively between the Naidoo and Ting studies does seem to show a difference in operative end points. Although the methods of measurement and reporting are different between the two studies, Naidoo and colleagues reported a 21.0-mm by 19.5-mm opening in contrast to a total mean area of 98.4 mm^2. Maximizing the extent of the neo-ostium carries little downside[40] and is a critical variable in the subjective and objective outcomes that the surgeon has the capability of influencing.[62]

Key Points

- Draf III is an effective way to salvage recalcitrant frontal sinusitis.
- Symptoms are improved in approximately 85% of patients.
- Although long-term patency rates vary, high patency rates (97%) are maintained and stable beyond 2 years in cases with large neo-ostia (20 mm × 20 mm).

SUMMARY

ESS is an effective intervention at improving QOL for patients with medically refractory CRS. The data supporting endoscopic Draf IIa frontal sinusotomy as part of ESS are limited to single institution case series. However, the data do demonstrate that most patients experience lasting frontal sinus patency on postoperative endoscopic examination and improvements in QOL. Salvage endoscopic frontal sinus surgery via a Draf III shows high rates of both neo-ostium patency and subjective improvements in symptoms at a 2-year time point. The long-term data are mixed and more study is warranted to establish the long-term efficacy at salvaging the most recalcitrant cases of frontal sinusitis.

REFERENCES

1. Soler ZM, Wittenberg E, Schlosser RJ, et al. Health state utility values in patients undergoing endoscopic sinus surgery. Laryngoscope 2011;121(12):2672–8.
2. Rudmik L, Smith TL, Schlosser RJ, et al. Productivity costs in patients with refractory chronic rhinosinusitis. Laryngoscope 2014;124(9):2007–12.
3. Rosenfeld RM, Piccirillo JF, Chandrasekhar SS, et al. Clinical practice guideline (update): adult sinusitis. Otolaryngol Head Neck Surg 2015;152(2 Suppl): S1–39.
4. Fokkens WJ, Lund VJ, Mullol J, et al. EPOS 2012: European position paper on rhinosinusitis and nasal polyps 2012. A summary for otorhinolaryngologists. Rhinology 2012;50(1):1–12.
5. Stammberger H, Posawetz W. Functional endoscopic sinus surgery. Concept, indications and results of the Messerklinger technique. Eur Arch Otorhinolaryngol 1990;247(2):63–76.
6. Timperley D, Schlosser RJ, Harvey RJ. Chronic rhinosinusitis: an education and treatment model. Otolaryngol Head Neck Surg 2010;143(5 Suppl 3):S3–8.
7. Chiu AG. Frontal sinus surgery: its evolution, present standard of care, and recommendations for current use. Ann Otol Rhinol Laryngol Suppl 2006;196:13–9.
8. Wormald PJ. Salvage frontal sinus surgery: the endoscopic modified Lothrop procedure. Laryngoscope 2003;113(2):276–83.
9. Draf W. Endonasal micro-endoscopic frontal sinus surgery: the Fulda concept. Operat Tech Otolaryngol Head Neck Surg 1991;2(4):234–40.

10. Smith TL, Litvack JR, Hwang PH, et al. Determinants of outcomes of sinus surgery: a multi-institutional prospective cohort study. Otolaryngol Head Neck Surg 2010; 142(1):55–63.

11. Gliklich RE, Metson R. Effect of sinus surgery on quality of life. Otolaryngol Head Neck Surg 1997;117(1):12–7.

12. Bhattacharyya N. Symptom outcomes after endoscopic sinus surgery for chronic rhinosinusitis. Arch Otolaryngol Head Neck Surg 2004;130(3):329–33.

13. Smith TL, Kern R, Palmer JN, et al. Medical therapy vs surgery for chronic rhino-sinusitis: a prospective, multi-institutional study with 1-year follow-up. Int Forum Allergy Rhinol 2013;3(1):4–9.

14. DeConde AS, Mace JC, Alt JA, et al. Comparative effectiveness of medical and surgical therapy on olfaction in chronic rhinosinusitis: a prospective, multi-institutional study. Int Forum Allergy Rhinol 2014;4:725–33.

15. DeConde AS, Mace JC, Alt JA, et al. Investigation of change in cardinal symptoms of chronic rhinosinusitis after surgical or ongoing medical management. Int Forum Allergy Rhinol 2015;5(1):36–45.

16. Naidoo Y, Wen D, Bassiouni A, et al. Long-term results after primary frontal sinus surgery. Int Forum Allergy Rhinol 2012;2(3):185–90.

17. DeConde AS, Suh JD, Mace JC, et al. Outcomes of complete vs targeted approaches to endoscopic sinus surgery. Int Forum Allergy Rhinol 2015;5(8):691–700.

18. Schaefer SD, Close LG. Endoscopic management of frontal sinus disease. Laryngoscope 1990;100(2 Pt 1):155–60.

19. Wigand ME, Hosemann WG. Endoscopic surgery for frontal sinusitis and its complications. Am J Rhinol 1991;5(3):85–9.

20. Moriyama H, Fukami M, Yanagi K, et al. Endoscopic endonasal treatment of ostium of the frontal sinus and the results of endoscopic surgery. Am J Rhinol 1994;8(2):67–70.

21. Christmas DA, Krouse JH. Powered instrumentation in dissection of the frontal recess. Ear Nose Throat J 1996;75(6):359–60, 363–4.

22. Jacobs JB. 100 years of frontal sinus surgery. Laryngoscope 1997;107(11 Pt 2): 1–36.

23. Hosemann W, Kühnel T, Held P, et al. Endonasal frontal sinusotomy in surgical management of chronic sinusitis: a critical evaluation. Am J Rhinol 1997;11(1):1–9.

24. Metson R, Gliklich RE. Clinical outcome of endoscopic surgery for frontal sinusitis. Arch Otolaryngol Head Neck Surg 1998;124(10):1090–6.

25. Wormald PJ. The axillary flap approach to the frontal recess. Laryngoscope 2002; 112(3):494–9.

26. Wormald PJ, Chan SZX. Surgical techniques for the removal of frontal recess cells obstructing the frontal ostium. Am J Rhinol 2003;17(4):221–6.

27. Chiu AG, Vaughan WC. Revision endoscopic frontal sinus surgery with surgical navigation. Otolaryngol Head Neck Surg 2004;130(3):312–8.

28. Chandra RK, Palmer JN, Tangsujarittham T, et al. Factors associated with failure of frontal sinusotomy in the early follow-up period. Otolaryngol Head Neck Surg 2004;131(4):514–8.

29. Friedman M, Bliznikas D, Vidyasagar R, et al. Long-term results after endoscopic sinus surgery involving frontal recess dissection. Laryngoscope 2006;116(4):573–9.

30. Chan Y, Melroy CT, Kuhn CA, et al. Long-term frontal sinus patency after endoscopic frontal sinusotomy. Laryngoscope 2009;119(6):1229–32.

31. Askar MH, Gamea A, Tomoum MO, et al. Endoscopic management of chronic frontal sinusitis: prospective quality of life analysis. Ann Otol Rhinol Laryngol 2015;124(8):638–48.

32. Abreu NA, Nagalingam NA, Song Y, et al. Sinus microbiome diversity depletion and *Corynebacterium tuberculostearicum* enrichment mediates rhinosinusitis. Sci Transl Med 2012;4(151):151ra124.

33. Bhandarkar ND, Mace JC, Smith TL. The impact of osteitis on disease severity measures and quality of life outcomes in chronic rhinosinusitis. Int Forum Allergy Rhinol 2011;1(5):372–8.

34. Soler ZM, Sauer D, Mace J, et al. Impact of mucosal eosinophilia and nasal polyposis on quality-of-life outcomes after sinus surgery. Otolaryngol Head Neck Surg 2010;142(1):64–71.

35. Valdes CJ, Bogado M, Samaha M. Causes of failure in endoscopic frontal sinus surgery in chronic rhinosinusitis patients. Int Forum Allergy Rhinol 2014;4(6): 502–6.

36. Macbeth R. The osteoplastic operation for chronic infection of the frontal sinus. J Laryngol Otol 1954;68(7):465–77.

37. Scott NA, Wormald P, Close D, et al. Endoscopic modified Lothrop procedure for the treatment of chronic frontal sinusitis: a systematic review. Otolaryngol Head Neck Surg 2003;129(4):427–38.

38. Weber R, Draf W, Keerl R, et al. Osteoplastic frontal sinus surgery with fat obliteration: technique and long-term results using magnetic resonance imaging in 82 operations. Laryngoscope 2000;110(6):1037–44.

39. Gross WE, Gross CW, Becker D, et al. Modified transnasal endoscopic Lothrop procedure as an alternative to frontal sinus obliteration. Otolaryngol Head Neck Surg 1995;113(4):427–34.

40. Chin D, Snidvongs K, Kalish L, et al. The outside-in approach to the modified endoscopic Lothrop procedure. Laryngoscope 2012;122(8):1661–9.

41. Gross CW, Zachmann GC, Becker DG, et al. Follow-up of University of Virginia experience with the modified Lothrop procedure. Am J Rhinol 1997;11(1): 49–54.

42. Casiano RR, Livingston JA. Endoscopic Lothrop procedure: the University of Miami experience. Am J Rhinol 1998;12(5):335–9.

43. Kikawada T, Fujigaki M, Kikura M, et al. Extended endoscopic frontal sinus surgery to interrupted nasofrontal communication caused by scarring of the anterior ethmoid: long-term results. Arch Otolaryngol Head Neck Surg 1999;125(1):92–6.

44. McLaughlin RB, Hwang PH, Lanza DC. Endoscopic trans-septal frontal sinusotomy: the rationale and results of an alternative technique. Am J Rhinol 1999; 13(4):279–87.

45. Ulualp SO, Carlson TK, Toohill RJ. Osteoplastic flap versus modified endoscopic Lothrop procedure in patients with frontal sinus disease. Am J Rhinol 2000;14(1):21–6.

46. Schulze SL, Loehrl TA, Smith TL. Outcomes of the modified endoscopic Lothrop procedure. Am J Rhinol 2002;16(5):269–73.

47. Schlosser RJ, Zachmann G, Harrison S, et al. The endoscopic modified Lothrop: long-term follow-up on 44 patients. Am J Rhinol 2002;16(2):103–8.

48. Samaha M, Cosenza MJ, Metson R. Endoscopic frontal sinus drillout in 100 patients. Arch Otolaryngol Head Neck Surg 2003;129(8):854–8.

49. Stankiewicz JA, Wachter B. The endoscopic modified Lothrop procedure for salvage of chronic frontal sinusitis after osteoplastic flap failure. Otolaryngol Head Neck Surg 2003;129(6):678–83.

50. Wormald PJ, Ananda A, Nair S. The modified endoscopic Lothrop procedure in the treatment of complicated chronic frontal sinusitis. Clin Otolaryngol Allied Sci 2003;28(3):215–20.

51. Khong JJ, Malhotra R, Selva D, et al. Efficacy of endoscopic sinus surgery for paranasal sinus mucocele including modified endoscopic Lothrop procedure for frontal sinus mucocele. J Laryngol Otol 2004;118(5):352–6.

52. Banhiran W, Sargi Z, Collins W, et al. Long-term effect of stenting after an endoscopic modified Lothrop procedure. Am J Rhinol 2006;20(6):595–9.

53. Tran KN, Beule AG, Singal D, et al. Frontal ostium restenosis after the endoscopic modified Lothrop procedure. Laryngoscope 2007;117(8):1457–62.

54. Shirazi MA, Silver AL, Stankiewicz JA. Surgical outcomes following the endoscopic modified Lothrop procedure. Laryngoscope 2007;117(5):765–9.

55. Nakagawa T, Ito J. Endoscopic modified Lothrop procedure for postoperative frontal mucocele. Acta Otolaryngol Suppl 2007;(557):51–4.

56. Eloy P, Vlaminck S, Jorissen M, et al. Type III frontal sinusotomy: surgical technique, indications, outcomes, a multi-university retrospective study of 120 cases. B-ENT 2011;7(Suppl 17):3–13.

57. Georgalas C, Hansen F, Videler WJM, et al. Long terms results of Draf type III (modified endoscopic Lothrop) frontal sinus drainage procedure in 122 patients: a single centre experience. Rhinology 2011;49(2):195–201.

58. Hildenbrand T, Wormald PJ, Weber RK. Endoscopic frontal sinus drainage Draf type III with mucosal transplants. Am J Rhinol Allergy 2012;26(2):148–51.

59. Naidoo Y, Bassiouni A, Keen M, et al. Long-term outcomes for the endoscopic modified Lothrop/Draf III procedure: a 10-year review. Laryngoscope 2014; 124(1):43–9.

60. Ting JY, Wu A, Metson R. Frontal sinus drillout (modified Lothrop procedure): long-term results in 204 patients. Laryngoscope 2014;124(5):1066–70.

61. Anderson P, Sindwani R. Safety and efficacy of the endoscopic modified Lothrop procedure: a systematic review and meta-analysis. Laryngoscope 2009;119(9): 1828–33.

62. Naidoo Y, Bassiouni A, Keen M, et al. Risk factors and outcomes for primary, revision, and modified Lothrop (Draf III) frontal sinus surgery. Int Forum Allergy Rhinol 2013;3(5):412–7.

Management of Frontal Sinus Cerebrospinal Fluid Leaks and Encephaloceles

Elisa A. Illing, MD, Bradford A. Woodworth, MD*

KEYWORDS

- Cerebrospinal fluid leak • Encephalocele • Frontal sinus • Anterior cranial base
- Skull base tumor • Endoscopic sinus surgery • Endoscopic skull base surgery

KEY POINTS

- Comprehensive preoperative workup including history, physical, imaging, and confirmatory laboratory testing will help determine the cause for cerebrospinal fluid leak or encephalocele.
- Hemostasis with topical and infiltrative vasoconstrictors aids in visualization and decreases risk of surgical error.
- Careful and complete exposure surrounding the encephalocele helps the surgeon control bleeding and permits greater working area.
- Aggressive postoperative antiemetics, stool softeners, and nasal packing support the repair against spikes in intracranial pressure in the early postoperative period.
- Vigilant postoperative endoscopy with debridement increases the chance of frontal sinus patency long-term.

 Video content accompanies this article at http://www.oto.theclinics.com.

INTRODUCTION

Traditional management of frontal sinus pathology (eg: trauma, neoplasms) involving the posterior table has primarily included the osteoplastic flap or cranialization procedures intended to obliterate or ablate the frontal sinus. However, recent developments in technical expertise, widespread frontal sinus training, and advancements in instrumentation now permit excellent surgical access to

Conflict of Interest/Financial Disclosures: B.A. Woodworth is a consultant for Smith and Nephew, Olympus, and Cook Medical.
Department of Otolaryngology, University of Alabama at Birmingham, BDB 563, 1720 2nd Avenue South, Birmingham, AL 35294, USA
* Corresponding author.
E-mail address: bwoodwo@hotmail.com

Otolaryngol Clin N Am 49 (2016) 1035–1050
http://dx.doi.org/10.1016/j.otc.2016.03.025

the frontal sinus posterior table using endoscopic approaches.[1–12] Mounting evidence indicates outcomes are equivalent to open techniques for eligible cases with the advantage of decreased morbidity and lack of external incisions. Skull base defects secondary to a variety of causes, including trauma, neoplasm, iatrogenic, congenital, and spontaneous pathology, may often be repaired using endoscopic techniques. The presence of cerebrospinal fluid (CSF) rhinorrhea indicates there is an open communication to the intracranial space, which places patients at risk for meningitis and other cerebral complications. To prevent these life-threatening sequelae, identification of the leak and repair of the associated defect is integral to appropriate management. Recognition of leaks preoperatively involves a high degree of clinical suspicion, imaging, laboratory testing, and nasal endoscopic examination. Careful surgical technique, individualized to each patient's pathology and anatomy, is vital to successful treatment and reducing the risk of postoperative complications, such as stenosis of the frontal recess, anosmia, intracranial hemorrhage, orbital complications, and persistence or recurrence of the CSF leak. The following discussion reviews pertinent frontal sinus anatomy, preoperative assessment, surgical techniques, types of repair, postoperative management, and published outcomes.

PREOPERATIVE PLANNING AND OUTCOMES

Preoperative evaluation should begin with a thorough history and physical examination, nasal endoscopy, and radiographic imaging. Patients will often describe constant or intermittent clear rhinorrhea associated with a salty or metallic taste and may complain of headaches from low or high (spontaneous CSF leaks from idiopathic intracranial hypertension) intracranial pressure (ICP). Additional symptoms reported with CSF leak or encephalocele may include unilateral or bilateral nasal obstruction, nausea, and neck stiffness. History of head trauma, prior sinus or neurologic surgery, congenital abnormalities, prior episodes of meningitis, and obesity should be assessed.

To identify the presence of a CSF leak, several diagnostic tools are available (**Table 1**). The invasiveness of the test and risks to patients with each of these tests should be considered carefully, as should the reported sensitivity and specificity of the test. Test characteristics depend significantly on the patient population studied, defect size, leak flow rate, and individual interpretation of results. Although a study may reveal the location of the leak, further investigation may be required during the surgery (discussed in surgical technique section) to definitively identify the location or assess for simultaneous leaks that may not have been detected during the original evaluation.

Surgical repair is generally indicated for all patients with active CSF leakage due to spontaneous, iatrogenic, and neoplastic causes to prevent intracranial infection. Conversely, for those with traumatic causes of CSF leak, bed rest and stool softeners are usually first-line therapy, as many leaks will close without further intervention. For those with congenital defects, surgical removal and repair is often indicated for children presenting with nasal obstruction from the intranasal encephalocele. Active CSF leak is less common, so observation for small, asymptomatic encephaloceles is a reasonable strategy.

Contraindications for skull base repair include patients with high risks of bleeding and severe medical comorbidities. Patients on anticoagulation or with low platelets from blood dyscrasias or disorders are at increased risk for intracranial hemorrhage. Careful consideration of holding anticoagulation in patients with cardiovascular

Table 1
Diagnostic tools for cerebrospinal fluid leak

Technique	Advantages	Disadvantages
Beta-2 transferrin	Noninvasive, accurate, patient can collect during intermittent episodes	Nonlocalizing
Computed tomography	Noninvasive, excellent bony detail, accessible	Cannot differentiate CSF from soft tissue, bony dehiscence/attenuation may be present without leak
Radioactive cisternogram	Localizes side of leak, utility for low and intermittent leaks	Imprecise localization, NOT recommended because of high-false positive rate[13]
CT cisternogram	Contrast may pool in frontal sinus, excellent bony detail	Invasive, not as diagnostic for intermittent leaks
MRI/cisternography	Excellent soft tissue detail to determine difference between CSF/brain/mucous, noninvasive	Poor bony detail
Intrathecal fluorescein	Precise localization, blue-light filter may increase sensitivity	Invasive, skull base exposure necessary for precise localization of leak, risks with high concentration or rapid injection

compromise should be discussed with the patients, families, and other medical care providers. Ideally, patients should not have concomitant infection of the paranasal sinuses; however, benefits of intervention usually outweigh the risks in the situation of an active CSF leak because of the danger of ascending infection. Repair should be performed with perioperative and continued postoperative culture-directed intravenous antibiotics with excellent CSF penetration. For patients undergoing planned repair for tumor resection or nonleaking encephalocele, attempts to clear the infection before surgery are recommended.

CAUSES

As part of a thorough history and physical and adjunct testing, the underlying cause of the CSF leak is usually identified, affecting many characteristics of the leak, including size and extent of bony dehiscence, degree of dural disruption, ICP, and meningoencephalocele formation. The main causes include trauma, neoplasm, and spontaneous and congenital defects.

Traumatic

Fractures of the frontal sinus are problematic, as there is an increased risk for late mucocele formation, intracranial injury, cosmetic deformity, and delayed CSF leak.[14] Approximately 5% to 12% of craniofacial injuries involve fractures of the frontal sinus from blunt or penetrating injuries, with the latter often causing significant comminution of the posterior table and greater chance of intracranial injury.[15] CSF leaks generally start within 48 hours to 3 months of the time of injury, although 5% may present in a more delayed fashion.[16] Although more than 70% of traumatic CSF leaks close with observation or conservative treatment, a 29% incidence of meningitis has been seen in long-term follow-up with nonsurgical management.[17] Severe fractures usually warrant surgical intervention because of a high risk of mucocele formation.[18] The complete clinical picture of patients, including stability and other comorbidities (facial fractures, orbital injuries, and so forth) must be considered in choosing a surgical approach that addresses both the CSF leak and minimizes the risk of mucocele formation.

Iatrogenic traumatic CSF leaks are most commonly caused by endoscopic sinus surgery and neurosurgical surgery. Inadequate knowledge of the anatomy, inappropriate use of powered instrumentation, and lack of preoperative evaluation of bony dehiscences are common features leading to surgical errors. The posterior table of the frontal sinus is much thinner and more fragile than the anterior table, especially when eroded by pressure from an expansile tumor or mucocele. During neurosurgery, CSF leaks may occur during a frontal craniotomy such that the superior or lateral recess is entered during removal of the bony plate. Leaks within the lateral frontal sinus are generally difficult to repair solely with an endoscopic approach and may require open osteoplastic flap or trephine assistance or ultimately a frontal sinus ablation or obliteration.

Neoplasm

Tumors of the anterior skull base can cause CSF leaks through direct erosion of the frontal recess and posterior table of the frontal sinus, by tumor regression after erosion (in response to chemotherapy or radiation) or as a result of surgical resection. CSF leaks may occur after planned reconstruction following intracranial, extracranial, or endoscopic resections of skull base tumors involving the posterior table for several reasons, including torn or devitalized flap repairs, retraction or insufficient size of flaps/grafts, and inadequate packing or support. Posterior table defects and frontal sinus floor defects (after cranialization) may still be present and contribute to CSF leak. Significant reduction in vascularity of the wound bed and/or healing from prior chemotherapy or radiation can also affect success rates.

Congenital

Congenital leaks and encephaloceles of the frontal sinus technically do not exist because the frontal sinus is not present at birth. However, congenital defects may be present within or adjacent to the frontal recess typically arising through a patent foramen cecum. Congenital skull base defects at the areas adjacent to the frontal recess may prove a significant challenge for repair, as many patients have low-lying skull bases and funnel-shaped defects.[11,19]

Spontaneous

If no other cause for CSF leak is identified, patients are labeled as having a spontaneous CSF leak. Spontaneous leaks frequently occur in obese middle-aged women with elevated ICP.[20] Over time, elevated ICP is thought to erode the skull base, producing the highest rate of encephalocele formation and recurrences following surgical repair compared with other causes.[21–23] The most common leak sites are from the cribriform plate, lateral recess of the sphenoid sinus, and posterior table of the frontal sinus.[9,24,25] Because of the high recurrence rate, adjuvant treatment to lower ICP is strongly recommended.[25]

FRONTAL SINUS ANATOMY

The frontal recess is defined anteriorly by the nasofrontal beak, laterally by the orbit, medially by the anterior attachment of the middle turbinate, and posteriorly by the ethmoid roof. There is significant anatomic variability regarding frontal recess cells, anterior-posterior diameter, and frontal sinus pneumatization, which can affect the choice of approach and reconstructive technique. CSF leaks of the frontal sinus are generally described as involving 3 areas: adjacent to the frontal recess, directly involving the frontal recess, and within the frontal sinus proper.[19] Skull base defects can span across these anatomic sites. Regardless of location, any endoscopic repair in these areas will require appropriate management of the frontal recess to prevent iatrogenic mucoceles or frontal sinusitis.

PATIENT POSITIONING

Before intubation, the surgeon should communicate with the anesthesia team to avoid positive pressure ventilation to prevent pneumocephalus. The authors recommend the endotracheal tube be secured with tape to the left lower lip, thus avoiding interference with the endoscopes and surgeon, who will position himself or herself at the patients' right side. Prophylactic antibiotic dosing before the start of the procedure is recommended, usually 2 g of ceftriaxone intravenously. In indicated cases, the neurosurgery team will place a lumbar drain, in which case patients will temporarily be in the right lateral decubitus position. Lumbar drains are typically used to instill fluorescein in patients with suspected elevated ICP (spontaneous CSF leaks), questionable defect site (some trauma), or for some large cranial base resections. Preservative-free 10% fluorescein (0.1 mL) is placed in 10 mL of the patients' own CSF or normal saline and slowly delivered via the drain over 10 minutes.[9] The patients are then returned to the supine position and temporarily placed in the Trendelenburg position to encourage circulation of the fluorescein intracranially. Image guidance may be calibrated at this point, and cotton pledgets with decongestant are placed in bilateral nasal cavities. Patients are then prepped and draped in the standard fashion.

PROCEDURAL APPROACH

The surgical goals for CSF leaks of the frontal sinus are to (1) successfully repair the leak and (2) allow for long-term patency of the frontal sinus or successful ablation or obliteration with meticulous removal of all mucosa from the frontal sinus. Surgical techniques to accomplish these goals are described next.

Endoscopic Approach

Endoscopic examination is performed first to evaluate the nasal anatomy and identify the location of the fluorescein stain if instilled by lumbar drain before the procedure. This site may be present on initial view or may be present only after better exposure is obtained. Once the leak site is identified, patients are placed in reverse Trendelenburg positioning to aid with hemostasis during the duration of the case, which begins with a full endoscopic sinus surgery on the affected side but may require middle turbinectomy or extended frontal procedures, such as the Draf III procedure, to obtain adequate exposure.

The endoscopic approach begins with standard maxillary antrostomy, ethmoidectomy, and sphenoidotomy. After the skull base is identified in the sphenoid, intervening partitions are removed in a posterior to anterior direction towards the frontal recess. Once at the frontal recess, the surgeon changes to a 70° endoscope, curved suction, and frontal sinus instrumentation to open the frontal sinus. Mucosal-sparing technique is used, such that only mucosa immediately around the defect is removed. If additional exposure is needed, the middle turbinate may be resected to repair defects that extend to the olfactory cleft. Extension to a Draf IIB frontal sinusotomy is usually required for unilateral defects (**Figs. 1** and **2**, Video 1), and a Draf III procedure may be performed for bilateral frontal sinus posterior table defects or for exposure of an anterior skull base tumor (**Fig. 3**, Video 2). The outside-in approach for Draf III has been described to decrease operating time[26] and may be applied in suitable cases and/or with an appropriate comfort level of the surgeon. Mucosal grafting of the anterior aspect of the frontal sinus can also decrease stenosis of the Draf III opening.[27]

For encephalocele cases, thorough bipolar electrocautery and/or a radiofrequency coblation (ArthroCare ENT, Sunnyvale, CA) device may be used once adequate exposure is obtained to reduce the encephalocele to the skull base[28] (**Fig. 4**, Video 3). Vigilant hemostasis is essential during reduction of the encephalocele, as dural or encephalocele vessels may retract and cause intracranial hemorrhage. Similarly, scrupulous removal of mucosa around the defect is necessary to prevent mucous secretion beneath the repair and encourage healing of the graft or flap.

Various grafting materials have been described in the literature, including fascia, fat, mucosa, allografts, xenografts, cartilage, bone grafts or pate, and dural substitute materials.[29] The authors almost universally use Biodesign porcine small intestinal submucosal (SIS) dural graft (Cook Medical, Bloomington, IN) for underlay and/or overlay grafting material. SIS graft offers several advantages, including no donor site morbidity, no swelling with hydration, and ease of handling without adhering to itself if crumpled or folded.[29] In cases with a large defect greater than 5 mm, elevated ICP, and sufficient epidural space, a septal or turbinate bone graft is used to further strengthen the repair. Bone grafting following tumor resection is not recommended, however, because of the large defect size (up to 5 cm) and possible need for adjuvant radiation.

To complete the multilayer repair, an overlay graft, usually of SIS material, or regular mucosal graft or flap is placed over the defect. The authors use a nasoseptal flap (NSF) if available, which can cover frontal sinus posterior table defects up to 3 cm in size depending on location within the sinus.[4] Fibrin sealant (Johnson & Johnson, Somerville, NJ) is used to tack the overlay graft or NSF into position, followed by an absorbable gelatin sponge to further support and secure the terrain of the repair. A 0.5-mm polymeric silicone stent is then placed in the frontal sinus outflow tract to prevent obstruction by repair material, followed by a nonlatex gloved cotton sponge (Medtronic, Jacksonville, FL) spacer inserted into the anterior aspect of the sphenoid sinus, extending just anterior to the frontal recess such that it fills the ethmoid cavity. Saline is then instilled into the spacer, resulting in its expansion; and a 2-0 polypropylene suture through the septum secures the spacer.

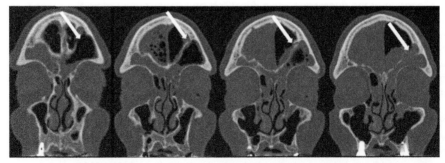

Fig. 1. Noncontrasted coronal computed tomography images of patient with a traumatic CSF leak after a fall. Arrow demonstrates the far lateral posterior table of frontal sinus fracture with associated pneumocephalus.

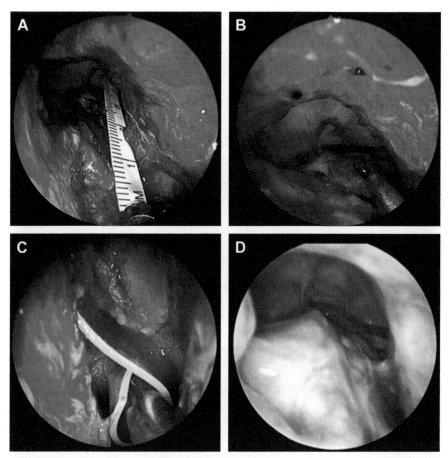

Fig. 2. (A) Intraoperative endoscopy using a 70° endoscope after Draf IIB procedure with measurement of 5-cm posterior table defect, (B) placement of SIS graft overlay, (C) placement of polymeric silicon sheeting frontal stent, and (D) postoperative endoscopy showing excellent healing of mucosa and frontal sinus patency.

Finally, if present and clamped, the lumbar drain is opened during emersion from anesthesia to prevent increases in ICP from Valsalva and coughing. Again, communication with the anesthesia team to perform topical laryngotracheal anesthesia before extubation, pretreatment with antiemetics, and avoidance of positive pressure mask ventilation is imperative to avoid preventable complications.

Extracranial Approach

Surgeons with limited equipment or endoscopic experience may consider open approaches to address frontal sinus encephaloceles or CSF leaks. Additionally, defects in the posterior table of the frontal sinus may not be completely addressed by an endoscopic approach, especially those in the lateral or superior aspect of the frontal sinus.[30] In some cases, a frontal trephine can be used to approach superior limits of the defect; however, if unable to meticulously remove mucosa from the defect area, an osteoplastic flap is recommended. The decision to graft and keep the frontal recess

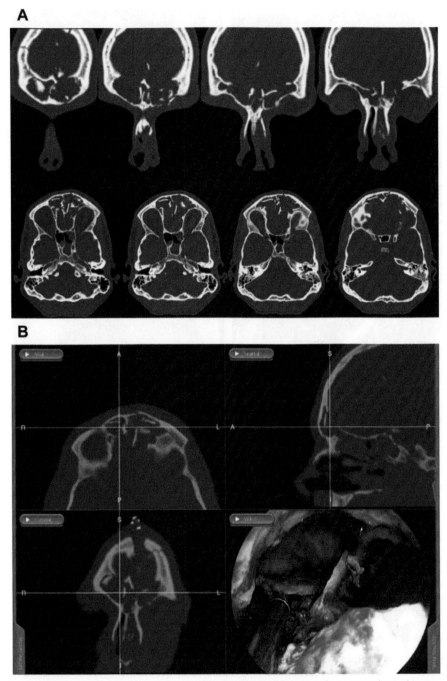

Fig. 3. (*A*) Coronal (*top*) and axial (*bottom*) noncontrasted computed tomography (CT) images of a patient with a self-inflicted gunshot wound with severely comminuted posterior table of the frontal sinus fracture. (*B*) Triplanar imaging with endoscopic, intraoperative view (*lower right*) with 70° endoscope view via a Draf III of the same patient. Note the posterior table bone fragment at the tip of the suction.

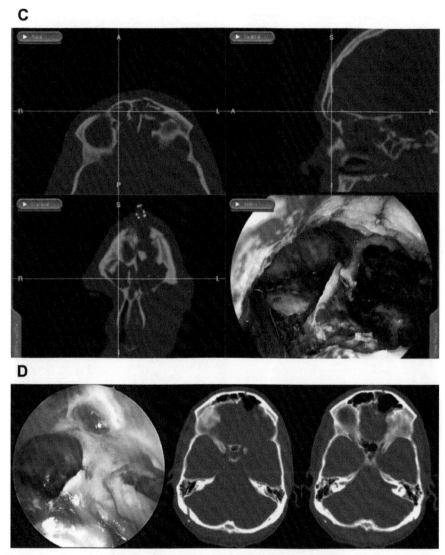

Fig. 3. (*continued*). (*C*) Triplanar imaging with endoscopic view (*lower right*) showing reduction of the bony fragment of the posterior table. (*D*) Postoperative endoscopy 6 weeks following surgery. A 70° endoscope in the frontal recess shows preservation of the frontal sinus with a small amount of absorbable gelatin sponge packing in place (*left*), with axial noncontrasted CT sinus demonstrating adequate reduction of fractures with purely endoscopic repair (*middle* and *right*). This patient did not have a nasal septal flap used in addition to his Biodesign underlay/overlay because of the involvement of the entire posterior table but has been without complication or sign of leak since his repair.

open or obliterate the sinus depends on the anatomy and comfort level of the surgeon. If nonobliterative, the surgeon must ensure that a patent frontal outflow tract exists to prevent remote mucocele formation and follow patients until healing to make sure the sinus stays patent.

A

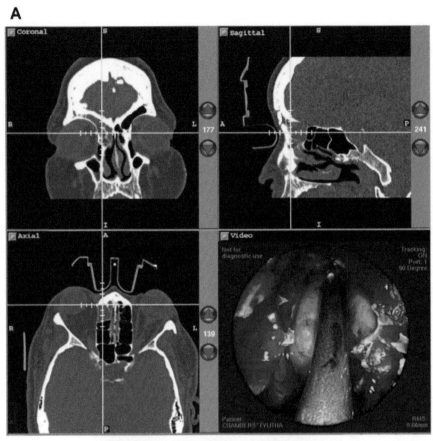

B

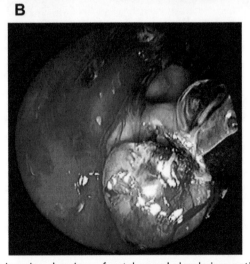

Fig. 4. (*A*) Triplanar imaging showing a frontal encephalocele in a patient with a previous extracranial approach to the defect, which failed to address the encephalocele or the patency of the frontal sinus. The right inferior image shows an endoscopic view of the encephalocele. (*B*) Endoscopic view of same patient demonstrating reduction of the encephalocele using the radiofrequency coblation device with a frontal sinus Draf IIB exposure.

C

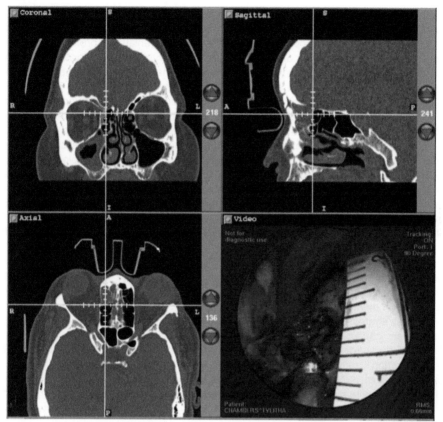

Fig. 4. (*continued*). (*C*) Triplanar imaging with endoscopic view (*bottom right*) following reduction of encephalocele with intraoperative measurements of the skull base defect.

The technique for performing an osteoplastic flap has been widely described,[31–33] with preparation of the defect site and grafting procedure similar to endoscopic management described earlier. If patency of the frontal outflow is not possible, obliteration should be performed. Stripping of all mucosa and drilling bony surfaces with a diamond burr is carefully performed, followed by underlay bone and overlay fascia grafts as indicated. Mucosa from the frontal recess is then stripped, and abdominal fat is placed in the sinus. Bilateral obliteration is recommended for small frontal sinuses or bilateral posterior table involvement.

Intracranial Approach

In severe cases of facial trauma or large anterior skull base neoplasms, significant frontal sinus posterior table defects are anticipated and likely best addressed by a craniotomy with cranialization of the frontal sinus and pericranial flap. Although excellent exposure is achieved, this approach does include a craniotomy and frontal lobe retraction. Possible postoperative complications include anosmia, intracranial hemorrhage, edema, epilepsy, and long-term memory issues.

POTENTIAL COMPLICATIONS AND MANAGEMENT

Despite careful technique and attention to patient anatomic and preoperative risk factors, complications may occur intraoperatively, immediately postoperatively, and in a delayed fashion. Intraoperatively, significant intracranial and orbital injury may occur. Attention to anatomy on imaging before surgery can identify potential areas of risk, including evading trauma to the anterior ethmoid artery and sphenopalatine arteries by avoiding extensive dissection in these areas if not involved in disease. Careful hemostasis with topical vasoconstrictors and minimizing mucosal trauma anteriorly aids optimal visualization. Careful hemostasis during reduction of the encephalocele helps prevent postoperative intracerebral hematoma. Should an orbital hematoma occur due to retraction of the anterior ethmoid artery, a lateral canthotomy and cantholysis should immediately be performed along with ophthalmologic consultation. With concerns for intracranial bleeding, urgent neurosurgical consultation is recommended. Careful hemostasis during surgery also lessens the risk of postoperative epistaxis. Hyposmia/anosmia may be prevented intraoperatively by avoiding excessive removal of the superior turbinate and careful dissection around olfactory fila. Counseling patients on loss of smell due to surgical intervention is imperative, if it is anticipated based on areas of pathology.

Postoperatively, anesthesia should avoid positive pressure mask ventilation to decrease risk of pneumocephalus. Careful monitoring in the perioperative period should also include close neurologic evaluation, with urgent imaging obtained for alteration in mental status or neurologic examination. Having patients on stool softeners and aggressive antiemetics, elevating the head of bed, and avoiding Valsalva maneuvers can prevent increases in ICP postoperatively that could result in early failure. If the surgeon is concerned for a postoperative CSF leak, prompt surgical re-exploration is recommended. Meningitis in this setting is rare; however, with persistent leak the risk is increased. Perioperative antibiotics and a watertight seal of the leak significantly decrease this risk. For patients with elevated ICP, consideration of oral acetazolamide or ventriculoperitoneal shunt is important to prevent recurrent or new CSF leaks.[25]

Delayed complications include frontal sinus stenosis, mucocele formation, or new or recurrent CSF leaks. Mucosal sparing techniques, postoperative stenting, vigilant in-office endoscopy with debridements, and maintenance with topical medications are helpful to maintain frontal sinus patency in the authors' experience. Early identification of narrowing is helpful, such that topical medications, such as steroids applied with nasal irrigations or in Mygind position may allow a nonoperative solution to narrowing. If these attempts fail, revision surgery may be pursued, with extended frontal sinus procedures, such as Draf III, considered. Mucocele formation can usually be addressed using an endoscopic approach. Remote, recurrent, or new-site CSF leaks are most common in patients with a spontaneous cause due to shunt failure or lack of appropriate ICP control. Revision surgery is required to address these new leaks, along with long-term control of elevated CSF pressure.

POSTPROCEDURAL CARE

Following surgery, patients are admitted for overnight observation in an intensive care unit setting for close observation and neurologic checks. A noncontrasted computed tomography scan of the head is obtained the morning following surgery to evaluate for cerebral hematoma or edema in cases of tumor resection, removal of large encephaloceles, or if neurologic alterations merit further investigation. For patients with elevated ICP, the lumbar drain is managed according to previously described

Table 2
Clinical results in the literature

Study, Year	Study Design	Study Groups	Clinical End Points
Woodworth & Schlosser,[19] 2005	Retrospective case series	Frontal CSF leaks treated endoscopically from 1998–2003	6 Patients with 7 frontal sinus CSF leaks; 3 spontaneous leaks, one congenital, one traumatic, and one iatrogenic: all repaired on primary attempt endoscopically
Jones et al,[4] 2012	Prospective case series	Frontal sinus CSF leaks treated over 3.5-y period by senior author	37 Patients included, various causes, initial successful endoscopic repair 91.9%, subsequent endoscopic repair success rate 97.3%, one patient required cranialization
Purkey et al,[5] 2009	Retrospective case series	Patients who underwent repair of supraorbital ethmoid CSF leaks from 2003–2007	8 Patients identified, most were obese, middle-aged women, with most patients having elevated ICP at time of surgery
Choi et al,[34] 2012	Retrospective case series	Patients treated for frontal sinus fractures over 10-y period	875 Patients identified, 68 had posterior table involvement, 11 had CSF leak; overall, 78% treated nonoperatively, 12% with ORIF with sinus preservation, 8% with obliteration, and 2% with cranialization
Chaaban et al,[14] 2012	Prospective case series	Patients treated from 2008–2012 with endoscopic repair of posterior table of frontal sinus fractures	13 Patients included, most requiring Draf IIb frontal sinusotomies, one with concomitant trephine, one required Draf III, only one required revision frontal sinusotomy
Gerbino et al,[15] 2000	Retrospective case series	Patients treated from 1987–1998 for fractures of the anterior and posterior tables of the frontal sinus	158 Patients included, 46 of which had comminuted and dislocated fractures of the posterior table, ± anterior table fractures were treated with bifrontal craniotomy and sinus cranialization, 3 of which died of meningitis, one had osteomyelitis, and 4 developed aesthetic frontal deformity

(continued on next page)

Table 2
(continued)

Study, Year	Study Design	Study Groups	Clinical End Points
Bhavana et al,[30] 2014	Retrospective case series	Patients with traumatic CSF rhinorrhea due to posterior table of frontal sinus fractures treated over 3 y	5 Patients identified and treated with trephine-assisted endoscopic repair with fat, bone graft, an fibrin glue, with all patients having successful primary repair at an average of 12-mo follow-up
Roehm & Brown,[12] 2011	Retrospective case series	Patients with frontal sinus CSF leak from a variety of causes repaired via unilateral endoscopic technique	4 Patients identified, with 3 successful repairs on primary attempt, one with communicating hydrocephalus requiring revision, 75% with frontal sinus patency, and 100% without leak at minimum 1-y follow-up

Abbreviation: ORIF, open reduction internal fixation.

protocol.[25] The authors only use diversion and CSF pressure monitoring for individuals suspected of having intracranial hypertension. All patients are maintained on intravenous antibiotics postoperatively for at least 24 hours and are transitioned to oral anti-staphylococcal antibiotics before discharge until nasal packing is removed during the clinic visit 9 to 13 days later. The authors find follow-up at this interval advantageous anecdotally as patients tend to experience less discomfort and bleeding. Patients are also placed on stool softeners, are aggressively treated for any nausea, and instructed on movement techniques to avoid Valsalva postoperatively. After initial follow-up, additional clinic visits are scheduled at 1- to 4-week intervals depending on concerns for ostial patency and postoperative healing issues (see **Table 1**).

OUTCOMES

Clinical outcomes on frontal sinus CSF leak management are listed in **Table 2**. Most publications on frontal sinus CSF leak and encephalocele repairs report a 90% or better repair rate, with patients having a spontaneous cause having greatest risk of surgical failure. In this patient population, regulation of intracranial hypertension via medical management (acetazolamide) or surgical diversion (ventriculoperitoneal shunt) is critical to successful management.[25]

SUMMARY

Frontal sinus encephaloceles and CSF leaks are increasingly addressed via endoscopic techniques; however, extracranial and intracranial approaches are necessary in some cases. Careful preoperative assessment of the disease cause and anatomic considerations will decrease the risk of intraoperative or postoperative complications.

SUPPLEMENTARY DATA

Supplementary data related to this article can be found at http://dx.doi.org/10.1016/j. otc.2016.03.025.

REFERENCES

1. Alexander NS, Chaaban MR, Riley KO, et al. Treatment strategies for lateral sphenoid sinus recess cerebrospinal fluid leaks. Arch Otolaryngol Head Neck Surg 2012;138(5):471–8.
2. Banks CA, Palmer JN, Chiu AG, et al. Endoscopic closure of CSF rhinorrhea: 193 cases over 21 years. Otolaryngol Head Neck Surg 2009;140(6):826–33.
3. Blount A, Riley K, Cure J, et al. Cerebrospinal fluid volume replacement following large endoscopic anterior cranial base resection. Int Forum Allergy Rhinol 2012; 2(3):217–21.
4. Jones V, Virgin F, Riley K, et al. Changing paradigms in frontal sinus cerebrospinal fluid leak repair. Int Forum Allergy Rhinology 2012;2(3):227–32.
5. Purkey MT, Woodworth BA, Hahn S, et al. Endoscopic repair of supraorbital ethmoid cerebrospinal fluid leaks. ORL J Otorhinolaryngol Relat Spec 2009; 71(2):93–8.
6. Schuster D, Riley KO, Cure JK, et al. Endoscopic resection of intracranial dermoid cysts. J Laryngol Otol 2011;125(4):423–7.
7. Woodworth BA, Neal JG, Schlosser RJ. Sphenoid sinus cerebrospinal fluid leaks. Op Tech Otolaryngol 2006;17:37–42.
8. Woodworth BA, Palmer JN. Spontaneous cerebrospinal fluid leaks. Curr Opin Otolaryngol Head Neck Surg 2009;17(1):59–65.
9. Woodworth BA, Prince A, Chiu AG, et al. Spontaneous CSF leaks: a paradigm for definitive repair and management of intracranial hypertension. Otolaryngol Head Neck Surg 2008;138(6):715–20.
10. Woodworth BA, Schlosser RJ. Repair of anterior skull base defects and CSF Leaks. Op Tech Otolaryngol 2006;18:111–6.
11. Woodworth BA, Schlosser RJ, Faust RA, et al. Evolutions in the management of congenital intranasal skull base defects. Arch Otolaryngol Head Neck Surg 2004;130(11):1283–8.
12. Roehm C, Brown SM. Unilateral endoscopic approach for repair of frontal sinus cerebrospinal fluid leak. Skull Base 2011;21(3):139–46.
13. Schlosser RJ, Bolger WE. Nasal cerebrospinal fluid leaks: critical review and surgical considerations. Laryngoscope 2004;114(2):255–65.
14. Chaaban MR, Conger B, Riley KO, et al. Transnasal endoscopic repair of posterior table fractures. Otolaryngol Head Neck Surg 2012;147(6):1142–7.
15. Gerbino G, Roccia F, Benech A, et al. Analysis of 158 frontal sinus fractures: current surgical management and complications. J Craniomaxillofac Surg 2000; 28(3):133–9.
16. Zlab MK, Moore GF, Daly DT, et al. Cerebrospinal fluid rhinorrhea: a review of the literature. Ear Nose Throat J 1992;71(7):314–7.
17. Bernal-Sprekelsen M, Bleda-Vazquez C, Carrau RL. Ascending meningitis secondary to traumatic cerebrospinal fluid leaks. Am J Rhinol 2000;14(4):257–9.
18. Guy W, Brissett AE. Contemporary management of traumatic fractures of the frontal sinus. Otolaryngol Clin North Am 2013;46(5):733–48.
19. Woodworth B, Schlosser RJ. Endoscopic repair of a congenital intranasal encephalocele in a 23 months old infant. Int J Pediatr Otorhinolaryngol 2005;69(7): 1007–9.

20. Schlosser RJ, Woodworth BA, Wilensky EM, et al. Spontaneous cerebrospinal fluid leaks: a variant of benign intracranial hypertension. Ann Otol Rhinol Laryngol 2006;115(7):495–500.

21. Gassner HG, Ponikau JU, Sherris DA, et al. CSF rhinorrhea: 95 consecutive surgical cases with long term follow-up at the Mayo Clinic. Am J Rhinol 1999;13(6): 439–47.

22. Hubbard JL, McDonald TJ, Pearson BW, et al. Spontaneous cerebrospinal fluid rhinorrhea: evolving concepts in diagnosis and surgical management based on the Mayo Clinic experience from 1970 through 1981. Neurosurgery 1985;16(3): 314–21.

23. Schick B, Ibing R, Brors D, et al. Long-term study of endonasal duraplasty and review of the literature. Ann Otol Rhinol Laryngol 2001;110(2):142–7.

24. Psaltis AJ, Schlosser RJ, Banks CA, et al. A systematic review of the endoscopic repair of cerebrospinal fluid leaks. Otolaryngol Head Neck Surg 2012;147(2): 196–203.

25. Chaaban M, Illing E, Riley KO, et al. Spontaneous cerebrospinal fluid leak repair: a five-year prospective evaluation. Laryngoscope 2014;124(1):70–5.

26. Chin D, Snidvongs K, Kalish L, et al. The outside-in approach to the modified endoscopic Lothrop procedure. Laryngoscope 2012;122(8):1661–9.

27. Conger BT Jr, Riley K, Woodworth BA. The Draf III mucosal grafting technique: a prospective study. Otolaryngol Head Neck Surg 2012;146(4):664–8.

28. Smith N, Riley KO, Woodworth BA. Endoscopic Coblator-assisted management of encephaloceles. Laryngoscope 2010;120(12):2535–9.

29. Illing E, Chaaban MR, Riley KO, et al. Porcine small intestine submucosal graft for endoscopic skull base reconstruction. Int Forum Allergy Rhinology 2013;3(11): 928–32.

30. Bhavana K, Kumar R, Keshri A, et al. Minimally invasive technique for repairing CSF leaks due to defects of posterior table of frontal sinus. J Neurol Surg B Skull Base 2014;75(3):183–6.

31. Goodale R, Montgomery WW. Anterior osteoplastic frontal sinus operation. Five years' experience. Otol Rhinol Laryngol 1961;70:860–80.

32. Goodale R, Montgomery WW. Technical advances in osteoplastic frontal sinusectomy. Arch Otolaryngol 1964;79:522–9.

33. Guggenheim P. Indications and methods for performance of osteoplastic-obliterative frontal sinusotomy with a description of a new method and some remarks upon the present state of the are of external frontal sinus surgery. Laryngoscope 1981;91:927–38.

34. Choi M, Li Y, Shapiro SA, et al. A 10-year review of frontal sinus fractures: clinical outcomes of conservative management of posterior table fractures. Plast Reconstr Surg. 2012;130(2):399–406.

Management of Frontal Sinus Tumors

Anne Morgan Selleck, MD[a], Dipan Desai, BS[a], Brian D. Thorp, MD[a], Charles S. Ebert, MD, MPH[a], Adam M. Zanation, MD[a,b,*]

KEYWORDS

- Frontal sinus • Tumor • Endoscopic • Sinonasal malignancy • Draf IIb • Draf III

KEY POINTS

- Accurate diagnosis of tumor type and appropriate staging are crucial to choosing the optimum management strategy.
- Considerations in determining the approach to frontal sinus tumors include frontal anatomy, tumor location, and tumor attachment sites.
- The endoscopic approaches to the frontal sinus include Draf IIa, IIb, and III procedures. These procedures are a continuum affording progressive access and exposure.
- The Draf IIb involves resection of the frontal sinus floor between the lamina papyracea and the nasal septum. The Draf III involves the bilateral removal of the frontal sinus floor through an anterosuperior septectomy, allowing confluence of the bilateral frontal sinuses.
- Although these tumors can often be approached via endoscopic techniques, surgeons should always be prepared to use open techniques.

OVERVIEW

Surgical management of frontal sinus tumors has traditionally challenged otolaryngologists because of the inherently narrow confines of the frontal sinus and its proximity to critical structures such as the anterior skull base, lamina papyracea, and anterior ethmoidal artery. Historically, removal of the various tumors that can occupy this space necessitated an open approach. After early and often morbid attempts at trephination and sinus obliteration, the use of osteoplastic flaps (OPFs), often with sinus obliteration, became the mainstay of surgical access to the frontal sinus.[1,2] Although

Conflict of interest: There are no conflicts of interest in the production of this article.

[a] Department of Otolaryngology—Head and Neck Surgery, University of North Carolina at Chapel Hill, 170 Manning Drive, CB #7070, Physician's Office Building, Room G-190, Chapel Hill, NC 27599-7070, USA; [b] Department of Neurosurgery, University of North Carolina at Chapel Hill, 170 Manning Drive, CB #7070, Physician's Office Building, Room G-190, Chapel Hill, NC 27599-7070, USA

* Corresponding author. 170 Manning Drive, CB #7070, Physician's Office Building, Room G-190, Chapel Hill, NC 27599-7070.
E-mail address: adam_zanation@med.unc.edu

this technique offered effective visualization and bimanual instrumentation, it too had the risk of morbidity or failure, including potential mucocele formation and loss of bone flap caused by chronic osteitis. Furthermore, long-term quality-of-life issues such as frontal bossing or depression and frontal neuralgia remained a possibility.[3–6] Through significant improvements in optical technologies and power instrumentation, the endonasal endoscopic approach has become a feasible and popular approach to a variety of paranasal sinus disorders. Many frontal sinus tumors can now be addressed with endoscopic techniques or via a combined approach.[2,7] Although endoscopic access to the frontal sinus can be complicated by the variability of frontal recess pneumatization, this approach offers significant advantages compared with previous open approaches. These advantages include decreased need for sinus obliteration, significantly easier postoperative monitoring, improved cosmetic results, and decreased morbidity. This article describes the most common tumors that affect the frontal sinus and discusses the current surgical approaches that best facilitate their removal.

PRIMARY TUMORS
Osteoma

Osteoma is the most common benign tumor of the paranasal sinuses, with a reported incidence of 0.5% to 3% in the general population.[8,9] These tumors are slow growing and are often discovered as an incidental finding.[10] Although osteomas were previously thought to occur most often in the frontal sinus, a recent study found that 55% of these tumors were located in the ethmoid sinuses, followed by the frontal sinuses at 37.5%.[11] Possibly because of their slow growth rate, most paranasal osteomas are asymptomatic and tend to only cause symptoms when they grow large enough to compress local structures or obstruct the sinus drainage pathways. Presenting symptoms can vary based on tumor location, but most frequently include frontal headache, facial pain, and chronic sinusitis.[10,12] Less commonly, these tumors can lead to the development of a mucocele or erode nearby structures such as the orbit or cranium.[13–16]

Because of their benign course, osteomas that are small and asymptomatic can be conservatively managed with observation.[12] However, specific indications for surgical intervention have been proposed. Savic and Djeric[17] recommended surgery for osteomas that are symptomatic, rapidly growing, obstructing the frontal recess, leading to rhinosinusitis, causing facial deformity, or extending beyond the frontal sinus (**Fig. 1**). More recently, Chiu and colleagues[18] proposed a frontal sinus osteoma grading system to guide decisions regarding appropriate surgical approach. Their system categorizes osteomas into 4 distinct grades based on 3 primary characteristics: the location of the base of attachment, anterior-posterior diameter of the lesion, and tumor location relative to a virtual sagittal plane through the lamina papyracea. Although their original recommendations for an endoscopic versus open approach based on these grades have been adjusted with subsequent endoscopic innovation, this grading system remains useful and is widely used in the literature.

Inverted Papilloma

Inverted papillomas (IP) are benign tumors of the paranasal sinuses. The incidence of IP has been reported at 0.74 per 100,000/y,[19] with 1% to 16% of these tumors originating in the frontal sinus[20] (**Fig. 2**). Overall, the most common site of origin for IP is the lateral nasal wall.[21,22] In addition, there seems to be a male predominance for these tumors, with a male to female ratio of 3.3:1.[20] IPs are typically treated with complete surgical resection because of their risk of recurrence without complete resection

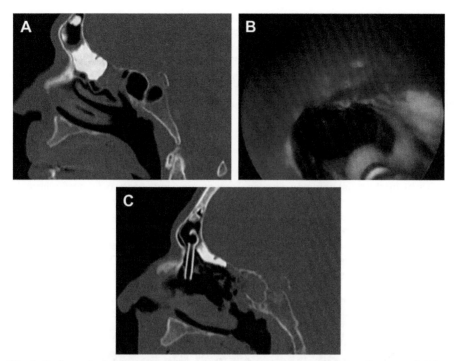

Fig. 1. Endoscopic drill-out of a frontal osteoma. (*A*) Sagittal image revealing an extensive frontal osteoma completely filling and obstructing the frontal outflow tract. (*B*) Progressive drill-out of the noted osteoma with access to the overlying frontal antrum allowing visualization of the margins of resection. (*C*) Postoperative imaging revealing subtotal resection of the noted osteoma with reestablishment of the frontal sinus outflow tract. Of note, because the patient presented with complications secondary to sinus obstruction, the goal of the procedure was to primarily reestablish a functional frontal sinus.

and potential to be locally destructive. Moreover, these lesions have the capacity to harbor or transform into squamous cell carcinoma (SCC). A recent meta-analysis of frontal sinus IP by Walgama and colleagues[20] discovered that 4.1% included SCC on final histopathology. This study also found that IPs of the frontal sinus are found

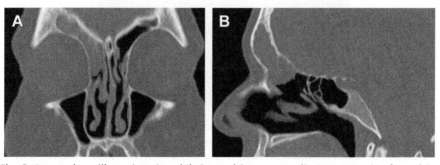

Fig. 2. Inverted papilloma imaging. (*A*) Coronal image revealing an extensive frontal inverted papilloma with appreciable hyperostosis about the roof of the frontal sinus. (*B*) Sagittal image revealing an extensive frontal inverted papilloma with appreciable hyperostosis about the posterior table. The noted hyperostosis indicates the region of tumor origin/attachment and should be evaluated when determining an appropriate approach.

bilaterally in about 16% of cases, a rate that is considerably greater than IP in other locations. This difference may be caused by incomplete initial resections or an intrinsic inability of the frontal intersinus septum to serve as an effective barrier to spread. One additional challenge with the removal of IPs is their tendency to recur. Walgama and colleagues[20] reported the rate of frontal sinus IP recurrence to be 22.4%, similar to previously reported rates of 22% and 16.7%.[23,24] These concerning findings show the importance of ensuring a complete resection when choosing among potential surgical approaches (**Fig. 3**).

SECONDARY TUMORS
Squamous Cell Carcinoma

SCC is by far the most common sinonasal malignancy and accounts for approximately 41% of such cancers. SCC occurs most frequently in the nasal cavity (46%) and maxillary sinus (40%), and least frequently in the frontal sinus.[25,26] Because initial symptoms can be vague and easily mistaken for benign sinonasal disease, SCC is typically diagnosed at advanced stages, and lymphatic metastasis is present in 10% to 20% of patients at the time of diagnosis[27,28] (**Fig. 4**). Thus, SCC carries a poor overall prognosis, with a reported 5-year survival rate of 50% to 60%.[29,30]

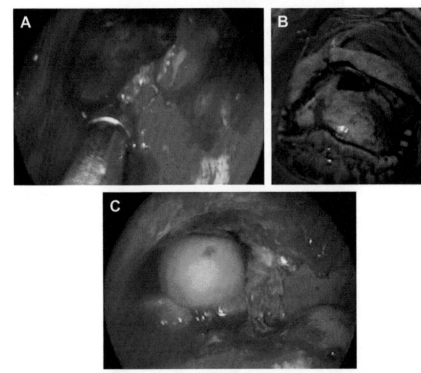

Fig. 3. Combined endoscopic and open approach to a frontal inverted papilloma. (*A*) Endoscopic approach and resection of the inverted papilloma with radiographic findings seen in **Fig. 2**. Note that a Draf IIb has been performed, allowing wide access to the frontal sinus antrum. (*B*) Open approach to the noted frontal inverted papilloma via a unilateral osteoplastic flap affording access to the posterior table and roof of the frontal sinus to ensure these sites of origin are adequately addressed. (*C*) Endoscopic view of the combined approach with a gloved finger seen traversing the site of the osteoplastic flap.

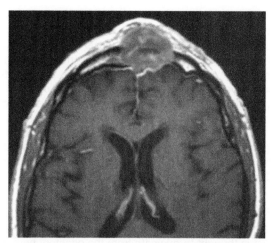

Fig. 4. Sinonasal squamous cell carcinoma imaging. Axial image revealing an extensive frontal sinonasal squamous cell carcinoma with frontal transgression and dural extension with associated lateral dural enhancement.

Occupational exposures to wood dust, nickel, or formaldehyde have been widely reported as risk factors for the development of both SCC and other sinonasal cancers.[31,32] These irritants may lead to carcinogenesis by eliciting chronic inflammation.[28] In addition, human papillomavirus has been linked to sinonasal SCC via malignant transformation of inverted papilloma tumors.[33] As with other sinonasal malignancies, surgical resection in adherence with oncologic principles with postoperative adjuvant therapies is the preferred mode of treatment. Depending on specific tumor extension and location, modern endoscopic approaches can effectively achieve complete resections of sinonasal SCC.

Sinonasal Undifferentiated Carcinoma

Sinonasal undifferentiated carcinoma (SNUC) is a rare and highly aggressive neuroendocrine malignancy that was first described by Frierson and colleagues[34] in 1986. The age-adjusted incidence is 0.02 per 100000, and there is a significant male predominance.[35,36] SNUC often initially presents with vague symptoms that worsen with rapid tumor growth. A literature review by Xu and colleagues[37] found that nasal obstruction, epistaxis, visual disturbances, and headache are the most common presenting symptoms. Previous studies have reported that most patients are diagnosed with advanced disease, with nearly 60% of patients having disease extending beyond the paranasal sinuses. Of those patients, 53% had orbital involvement, 41% had skull base involvement, and 13% had brain involvement.[38] Distant metastasis to the neck, lungs, liver, and bone has also been reported. The long-term prognosis at the time of SNUC diagnosis is grim, with a reported median survival of 22.1 months and a 5-year survival of 34.9%.[35] Because of this high mortality, SNUC has been treated with a variety of multimodal approaches, including aggressive surgical resection when possible plus adjuvant and/or induction chemotherapy and/or radiation. Further research is required to elucidate the optimum treatment regimen for these aggressive carcinomas.

Small Cell Neuroendocrine Carcinoma

Small cell neuroendocrine carcinomas (SNECs) are poorly differentiated, aggressive malignancies that predominantly occur in the lung. However, approximately 4% of

SNECs occur in extrapulmonary sites, including the paranasal sinuses.[39] Of note, all SNEC tumors share similar histologic features. Detailed morphologic and immunohistochemical analysis is crucial for accurate diagnosis and to distinguish these malignancies from other sinonasal neuroendocrine malignancies, namely SNUC and esthesioneuroblastoma.[40] As with SNUC, patients with SNEC often present with advanced disease, in part because of similar, nonspecific presenting symptoms, such as epistaxis, nasal obstruction, and nasal discharge. Overall, because of a combination of late presentation and their shared characteristics with pulmonary SNEC, sinonasal SNECs may be reasonably treated first with a chemotherapy or radiotherapy regimen, with surgical intervention reserved primarily for nonresponders.[41,42] Despite these interventions, the rates of local recurrence and metastasis are each approximately 30% and the 5-year survival is only 10%.[40]

Esthesioneuroblastoma

Esthesioneuroblastoma (ENB), also referred to as olfactory neuroblastoma, is a sinonasal neoplasm that is thought to originate from the olfactory neuroepithelium of the superior nasal cavity. ENB is rare and accounts for 3% to 6% of sinonasal malignancies.[43] Although it was previously thought to be a low-grade malignancy, it is now known that ENB commonly invades local structures, including the paranasal sinuses, cranial vault, and orbit, and has a propensity for distant metastases. As with the previously discussed SNEC and SNUC, proper histology and immunologic analysis are crucial to avoiding misdiagnosis, which can lead to selection of inappropriate treatment plans.[40,44] Cohen and colleagues[45] showed this potential hazard after reviewing previously diagnosed ENB at their institution and finding that 10 out of 12 of these tumors carried an incorrect diagnosis. The rarity of this tumor has largely limited the literature to retrospective studies and an ideal treatment method has been difficult to elucidate. In the past, a craniofacial resection with adjuvant radiation was the gold standard of treatment,[46] but endoscopic resection is now possible and preferred for certain patients in whom proper oncological principles are feasible. A large meta-analysis by Devaiah and Andreoli[47] found no difference in survival rate between surgical approaches, a finding also corroborated by Tajudeen and colleagues.[48] Overall, the combined approach of surgical resection with radiotherapy and possible chemotherapy seems to be the appropriate treatment modality for most patients with ENB.[44,49-51] Of note, ENB tumors have shown a prolonged time to both local recurrence and distant metastasis, and proper management necessitates long-term follow-up for periods even greater than 10 years.[49,52,53]

Sinonasal Non-Hodgkin Lymphoma

Mature B-cell non-Hodgkin lymphoma (NHL), which includes diffuse large B-cell NHL, is the second most common sinonasal malignancy after SCC. As a group, these tumors comprise approximately 10% of all sinonasal malignancies and are found most frequently in the maxillary sinus and nasal cavity, at 36.9% and 34.0%, respectively.[26] These malignancies may have similar clinical presentations to other tumors of this region and typically cause symptoms via mass effect. However, sinonasal mature B-cell NHL may also have symptoms that are more specific to B-cell lymphomas, namely fever and weight loss.[54] These malignancies have a reported 5-year disease-specific survival of 63.5% to 68.0%, which compares favorably with survival rates of other sinonasal malignancies.[26,55] Surgery serves virtually no role in the management of non-Hodgkin lymphoma, and these malignancies are primarily treated with a combination of chemotherapy and radiation therapy.[56]

SPECIAL CONSIDERATIONS: PEDIATRIC PATIENTS

Frontal sinus development in pediatric patients significantly affects surgical management. At birth, the frontal sinus is typically absent. The frontal sinus is the last of the paranasal sinuses to form and generally begins to pneumatize at age 2 years when the anterior-most ethmoid cell merges with the frontal bone. This nascent frontal sinus continues to grow vertically and is fairly well formed by age 8 years. However, it continues to undergo further development until age 20 years. These anatomic differences are important to consider when treating pediatric patients.

PREOPERATIVE PLANNING AND PREPARATION

Once the decision is made to surgically remove a frontal sinus tumor, the first surgical decision in the planning process is to determine the approach. There are 3 broad categories of surgical approaches to a frontal sinus tumor: open, endoscopic, or a combined approach. In order to make this decision, a computed tomography scan, compatible with intraoperative navigational systems, of the sinuses is essential.

Frontal sinus dimensions and anatomy are among the initial considerations in the ability to perform an endoscopic resection.[18] According to Draf,[57] the endoscopic Draf III procedure requires a frontal sinus to have an anterior to posterior diameter of at least 0.8 cm in order for the procedure to be technically possible. Sieśkiewicz and colleagues[58] stated that an anterior to posterior diameter of the frontal sinus less than 10 mm is a contraindication to an endoscopic approach. Sieśkiewicz and colleagues[58] also stated that increased convexity of the posterior wall of the frontal sinus also makes tumor removal difficult, because a more pronounced convexity minimizes the ability of endoscopic instruments to reach the attachment of the tumor. The size of the tumor relative to the frontal sinus also needs to be considered. It should also be noted that frontal sinus tumors limit the amount of space that is available for instruments to be able to access the space and manipulate the tumor.[18]

The tumor's location is also an important factor. The frontal sinus can be difficult to access, so tumors located laterally or with extensive lateral spread are considered by some clinicians to be a contraindication to an entirely endoscopic approach.[58] A Draf III should be considered in these tumors because it allows for an improved angle of visualization and the ability to maneuver instrumentation into the more lateral corners of the frontal sinus. Tumors located behind the virtual plane of the lamina papyracea are also proposed by some investigators as being more difficult to remove endoscopically.[58] The site of attachment is another important consideration, because those tumors with a superior attachment to the posterior wall of the sinus can be difficult to access.[58] Tumors attached to the lower half of the posterior wall of the frontal sinus are much easier to approach endoscopically.[59] Walgama and colleagues[20] reviewed frontal sinus inverting papillomas and found that tumors with a posterior wall attachment had the lowest recurrence rate (0%), although this rate was not statistically significant compared with other subsites ($P = .51$).

Another consideration that should be included in the discussion of surgical approach is the length of surgical time.[2] Although endoscopic cases in general can be prolonged compared with open procedures, surgical time can be particularly prolonged in cases of solid ivory-type osteomas given that the endoscopic disposable burrs tend to break frequently during removal.[60] Surgical time can become a significant contributor to the decision of surgical approach, especially given certain patient comorbidities.

Frontal sinus osteomas deserve special mention, because the grading system created by Chiu and colleagues[18] has helped establish endoscopic guidelines. Chiu and colleagues[18] studied 9 frontal sinus osteomas and decided that the endoscopic limit for frontal sinus osteomas was a grade II osteoma; III and IV had to be approached in an open fashion given the risk of cerebrospinal fluid (CSF) leak and inability to fully access the tumor to allow total resection. A study by Seiberling and colleagues[60] examined 25 cases of frontal sinus osteoma, of which 6 were grade III and 10 were classified as grade IV. Of this cohort, 2 of the grade III and IV patients underwent OPF procedures, and the rest were approached via a Draf III. Importantly, 2 of the grade IV patients undergoing the Draf III required an additional approach for tumor removal, which highlights the potential need for a combined approach in higher-grade tumors. The investigators concluded that grade III and IV osteomas could be approached endoscopically with a Draf III, although this approach was balanced with the increased risk of residual tumor and stenosis of the frontal sinus neo-ostium. Ledderose and colleagues[59] also examined 24 patients with a frontal sinus osteoma, 16 of whom had a grade III or IV osteoma. Of the 16 patients, 3 could be approached completely endoscopically, 4 required an open approach, and the remaining cohort were approached through a combination endoscopic and open approach. The investigators stated that the use of an intraoperative navigation system made a significant difference in their ability to approach tumors endoscopically. Before the use of navigational systems, they were unable to approach any tumor solely endoscopically. Rokade and Sama[2] discussed factors that they thought made endoscopic removal of osteomas difficult, including, "grade III and IV osteomas that occupy more than 75% of the frontal sinus, significant posterior table erosion, presenting with previous meningitis or CSF leak, extensive intracranial extension, and a significant supraorbital component with lateral orbital mucoceles"[2] (**Fig. 5**). These studies highlight the importance of the grading system, emphasize the increased difficulty in removing higher (III and IV) grade osteomas, and potential other factors to consider regarding the osteoma.

With regard to the inverting papilloma, total surgical resection is of paramount concern in order to prevent recurrence and local destruction, and to survey the tumor for SCC. Walgama and colleagues[20] reviewed 11 studies with a total of 49 patients who had frontal sinus inverting papilloma. They found the following incidence of surgical approach: 42.9% had a Draf II, 20.4% had a Draf III, 26.5% had an osteoplastic flap, and 10.2% had an endoscopic frontal trephination combined with an additional endoscopic approach. The recurrence rate was 22.4% for all approaches and no statistically significant difference was seen between the approaches. The lack of difference between the recurrence rates indicates the comparable ability of the endoscopic approach to provide total resection compared with the traditional open approach. However, the high rate of recurrence of the inverting papilloma in the frontal sinus speaks to the difficulty of resection in this area.[20]

Another consideration with regard to the surgical approach is surgeon skill and experience. The endoscopic approach requires an experienced surgeon given that these tumors are a rare clinical entity.[59]

Before surgery the patient can be started on topical or systemic steroids in order to minimize vascularity and edema. This treatment can allow decreased bleeding and thus improved visibility during the procedure.[61]

PROCEDURAL APPROACH

There are several endoscopic approaches to a frontal sinus tumor, including Draf IIa, IIb, and III approaches. These procedures are on a continuum, allowing increasing access and visualization of the frontal sinus. Once the frontal sinus has been approached

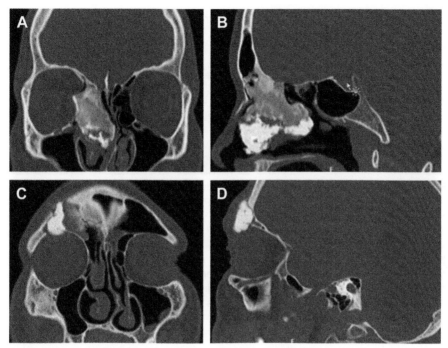

Fig. 5. Osteoma imaging. (*A, B*) Coronal and sagittal images revealing an extensive right frontal osteoma with sinonasal and orbital extension. Given the position of the osteoma and absence of significant lateral extension this lesion was amenable to endoscopic resection. (*C, D*) Coronal and sagittal images revealing an extensive right frontal osteoma with superolateral extension about the roof of the frontal sinus. Given the position of the osteoma and significant lateral extension this lesion was amenable to an open approach for resection.

and opened the tumor's attachment site can be localized and the tumor can be removed. These procedures are conducted under general anesthesia with the patient in a supine position. When used, a navigation system is always set up before surgery. Topical vasoconstrictors and 1% lidocaine with epinephrine are used at the discretion of the surgeon.

Regardless of the approach used, there are several key points to be remembered in frontal sinus surgery. Identification and awareness of the posterior limit of the frontal sinus is essential to decrease the risk of injury to the skull base.[62] In addition, visualization of the tumor attachment site is critical, because this allows safe and total removal.[58]

Surgery on the frontal sinus, unless completed previously, is preceded by an ethmoidectomy, including comprehensive dissection of the agger nasi region and associated frontal cells.[57]

Following the noted dissections, the determined frontal approach can be performed. A Draf IIa procedure involves removal of the ethmoidal cells protruding into the frontal sinus. The floor of the frontal sinus between the lamina papyracea and the middle turbinate is resected. This approach is limited for the use of tumors because the exposure is minimal. The Draf IIb, also known also the unilateral frontal sinus drill-out, involves an extended resection of the frontal sinus floor between the lamina papyracea and the nasal septum[63] (**Figs. 6** and **7**). A Draf III, also known as

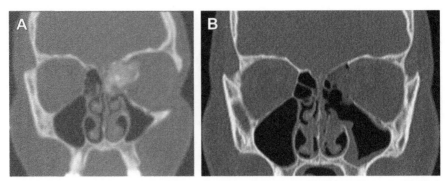

Fig. 6. Left orbitofrontal osteoma. (*A*) Preoperative coronal image revealing a left orbitofrontal osteoma without significant lateral or superior orbital extension. (*B*) Postoperative coronal image revealing gross total resection following an endoscopic resection.

the endoscopic modified Lothrop approach, provides maximal access by bilateral removal of the frontal sinus floor and the anterosuperior nasal septum, providing an orbit-to-orbit exposure.[63] This procedure was initially described in 1914 as an external technique and it was not until 1991 that it was adapted as an endoscopic transnasal approach.[2]

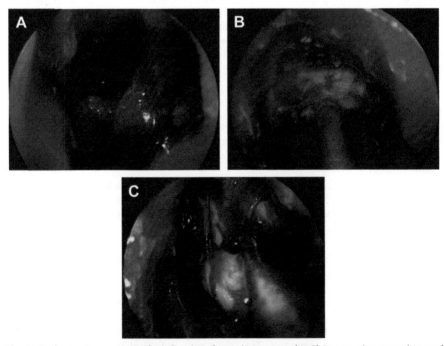

Fig. 7. Endoscopic resection of a left orbitofrontal osteoma. (*A, B*) Progressive resection and drill-out of the noted osteoma. As the margins of dissection are identified, the frontal outflow tract is widely opened. (*C*) Following extensive drill-out the remaining osteoma about the lamina papyracea is meticulously dissected and removed en bloc.

There are several additional considerations that must be kept in mind during an endoscopic approach to a frontal sinus tumor. Depending on the size and location of the tumor, it can potentially completely fill the middle meatus and obstruct access to the frontal recess.[64] Drilling with a burr can become a significant challenge when the tumor completely fills the frontal recess. The frontal sinus anatomy and boundaries can also be difficult to recognize if the tumor obstructs the potential margins of dissection, which also increase the risk to the orbit and skull base given how difficult it is for the surgeon to fully visualize the anatomic boundaries of the frontal sinus.[64]

POTENTIAL COMPLICATIONS AND MANAGEMENT

The important structures surrounding the frontal sinus include the lamina papyracea, cribriform plate, skull base, and anterior ethmoidal artery. Complications can occur if these structures are violated during the course of surgery. Orbital entry can potentially lead to injury to the eye, ocular muscles, and/or the optic nerve. Bleeding can result from injury to the anterior ethmoidal artery, leading to intranasal bleeding or intraorbital bleeding and resulting in a retro-orbital hematoma, which is a surgical emergency. Intracranial or skull base violation may result in a CSF leak, which must be immediately identified and repaired.

Often with the Draf III procedure the mucosa of the anterior and lateral walls of the frontal sinus is removed, leading to osteoneogenesis, scarring, and subsequent stenosis or closure of the ostium.[65] A study by Seiberling and colleagues[60] found that 5 out of 14 patients who underwent a Draf III procedure for frontal sinus osteoma had significant narrowing of the frontal ostium. A review of Draf III procedures, performed for tumor, chronic rhinosinusitis, and trauma, in 18 studies involving 612 patients, found that 19% of patients had stenotic or closed frontal sinus ostia.[65] Conger and colleagues[65] discussed a method for mucosal grafting in order to prevent stenosis. Septal mucosa was harvested from the septectomy in the initial stage of the Draf III procedure and was then positioned over the exposed bone in the anterior and lateral positions. All 27 patients studied, 14 of whom had a frontal sinus tumor, had a successful procedure with less than a 50% reduction in diameter of the frontal sinus ostia.

POSTPROCEDURAL CARE AND RECOVERY

Following surgery, it has been found that hospitalization times are decreased in those patients undergoing endoscopic procedures. Ledderose and colleagues[59] examined hospitalization time after surgical removal of frontal sinus osteomas, and found an average stay of 9.2 days for open approaches versus an average of 5.3 days for endoscopic approaches.

Postoperative management is crucial for good surgical outcome. Patients are often given postoperative courses of oral antibiotics of varying duration at the surgeon's discretion.[62] Patients are instructed to do saline irrigations at least 4 to 6 times a day. Patients are seen between 7 to 14 days postoperatively in the clinic for an endoscopic examination and removal of crusts and adhesions. Subsequent follow-up is dictated by endoscopic findings, degrees of healing, and surgeon preference.[62]

OUTCOMES

Recurrence is a common concern with tumor removal. Seiberling and colleagues[60] found that, in 4 of their endoscopic cases, 5% to 10% of residual tumor was left at the osteoma attachment site to the skull base. However, at an average follow-up of 60 months, no recurrence was found in these cases. It is thought that the lack of recurrence is secondary to the pattern of growth of the osteoma.[66] It is thought that the growth center of osteomas is centrally located, so by removing the central portion growth ceases.[66] However, there are reports in the literature of the recurrence of osteomas when full resection is not achieved.[67] Walgama and colleagues[20] did a systematic review of 49 cases of inverted papilloma of the frontal sinus that had an overall recurrence rate of 22.4%. They also examined the rate of recurrence based on surgical approach. Recurrence rates for Draf II, Draf III, osteoplastic flap, and endoscopic frontal trephination were respectively 23.8%, 30%, 15.4%, and 20%. They found no statistically significant difference between the 4 surgical approaches.

Outcome data regarding postoperative function or symptoms are sparse. Ledderose and colleagues[59] examined their 19 patients with frontal sinus osteoma and administered a postoperative SNOT-20 (Sino-Nasal Outcome Test 20) quality-of-life survey, providing some information regarding postoperative change and subjective assessment of outcome. These results were not separated by surgical approach, making it difficult to assess the subjective outcome difference attributable to surgical approach. Further study is needed in this area.

SUMMARY

With the advent of the Draf procedures and ever-improving surgical tools the endoscopic approach has become increasingly feasible for the management of frontal sinus tumors. Despite these advancements, frontal sinus anatomy in concert with tumor characteristics can make endoscopic removal difficult and surgeons should also be versed in open approaches. Although there is literature on the more common tumors of the frontal sinus, including inverting papilloma and osteoma, there is a paucity of data on the remaining tumors and associated outcomes. Further study is essential to further advance endoscopic treatment of frontal sinus tumors.

REFERENCES

1. Goodale RL, Montgomery WW. Five years' experience with the osteoplastic frontal sinus operation. Laryngoscope 1961;71(12):1584–5.
2. Rokade A, Sama A. Update on management of frontal sinus osteomas. Curr Opin Otolaryngol Head Neck Surg 2012;20(1):40–4.
3. Catalano PJ, Lawson W, Som P, et al. Radiographic evaluation and diagnosis of the failed frontal osteoplastic flap with fat obliteration. Otolaryngol Head Neck Surg 1991;104(2):225–34.
4. Correa AJ, Duncavage JA, Fortune DS, et al. Osteoplastic flap for obliteration of the frontal sinus: five years' experience. Otolaryngol Head Neck Surg 1999; 121(6):731–5.
5. Weber R, Draf W, Keerl R, et al. Osteoplastic frontal sinus surgery with fat obliteration: technique and long-term results using magnetic resonance imaging in 82 operations. Laryngoscope 2000;110(6):1037–44.
6. Alsarraf R, Kriet J, Weymuller EA Jr. Quality-of-life outcomes after osteoplastic frontal sinus obliteration. Otolaryngol Head Neck Surg 1999;121(4):435–40.
7. London SD, Schlosser RJ, Gross CW. Endoscopic management of benign sinonasal tumors: a decade of experience. Am J Rhinol 2002;16(4):221–7.
8. Broniatowski M. Osteomas of the frontal sinus. Ear Nose Throat J 1984;63(6): 267–71.
9. Earwaker J. Paranasal sinus osteomas: a review of 46 cases. Skeletal Radiol 1993;22(6):417–23.

10. Smith ME, Calcaterra TC. Frontal sinus osteoma. Ann Otol Rhinol Laryngol 1989; 98(11):896–900.
11. Erdogan N, Demir U, Songu M, et al. A prospective study of paranasal sinus osteomas in 1,889 cases: changing patterns of localization. Laryngoscope 2009; 119(12):2355–9.
12. Lund VJ, Stammberger H, Nicolai P, et al. European position paper on endoscopic management of tumours of the nose, paranasal sinuses and skull base. Rhinol Suppl 2010;(22):1–143.
13. Jurlina M, Janjanin S, Melada A, et al. Large intracranial intradural mucocele as a complication of frontal sinus osteoma. J Craniofac Surg 2010;21(4):1126–9.
14. Akay KM, Onguru O, Sirin S, et al. Association of paranasal sinus osteoma and intracranial mucocele—two case reports. Neurol Med Chir (Tokyo) 2004;44(4): 201–4.
15. Tsai CJ, Ho CY, Lin CZ. A huge osteoma of paranasal sinuses with intraorbital extension presenting as diplopia. J Chin Med Assoc 2003;66(7):433–5.
16. Summers LE, Mascott CR, Tompkins JR, et al. Frontal sinus osteoma associated with cerebral abscess formation: a case report. Surg Neurol 2001;55(4):235–9.
17. Savic DL, Djeric DR. Indications for the surgical treatment of osteomas of the frontal and ethmoid sinuses. Clin Otolaryngol Allied Sci 1990;15(5):397–404.
18. Chiu AG, Schipor I, Cohen NA, et al. Surgical decisions in the management of frontal sinus osteomas. Am J Rhinol 2005;19(2):191–7.
19. Buchwald C, Franzmann MB, Tos M. Sinonasal papillomas: a report of 82 cases in Copenhagen County, including a longitudinal epidemiological and clinical study. Laryngoscope 1995;105(1):72–9.
20. Walgama E, Ahn C, Batra PS. Surgical management of frontal sinus inverted papilloma: a systematic review. Laryngoscope 2012;122(6):1205–9.
21. Krouse JH. Endoscopic treatment of inverted papilloma: safety and efficacy. Am J Otolaryngol 2001;22(2):87–99.
22. Weissler MC, Montgomery WW, Turner PA, et al. Inverted papilloma. Ann Otol Rhinol Laryngol 1986;95(3 Pt 1):215–21.
23. Yoon BN, Batra PS, Citardi MJ, et al. Frontal sinus inverted papilloma: surgical strategy based on the site of attachment. Am J Rhinol Allergy 2009;23(3):337–41.
24. Dubin MG, Sonnenburg RE, Melroy CT, et al. Staged endoscopic and combined open/endoscopic approach in the management of inverted papilloma of the frontal sinus. Am J Rhinol 2005;19(5):442–5.
25. Turner JH, Reh DD. Incidence and survival in patients with sinonasal cancer: a historical analysis of population-based data. Head Neck 2012;34(6):877–85.
26. Dutta R, Dubal PM, Svider PF, et al. Sinonasal malignancies: a population-based analysis of site-specific incidence and survival. Laryngoscope 2015;125(11): 2491–7.
27. Bhattacharyya N. Cancer of the nasal cavity: survival and factors influencing prognosis. Arch Otolaryngol Head Neck Surg 2002;128(9):1079–83.
28. Llorente JL, Lopez F, Suarez C, et al. Sinonasal carcinoma: clinical, pathological, genetic and therapeutic advances. Nat Rev Clin Oncol 2014;11(8):460–72.
29. Lee CH, Hur DG, Roh HJ, et al. Survival rates of sinonasal squamous cell carcinoma with the new AJCC staging system. Arch Otolaryngol Head Neck Surg 2007;133(2):131–4.
30. Sanghvi S, Khan MN, Patel NR, et al. Epidemiology of sinonasal squamous cell carcinoma: a comprehensive analysis of 4994 patients. Laryngoscope 2014; 124(1):76–83.

31. Klein RG, Schmezer P, Amelung F, et al. Carcinogenicity assays of wood dust and wood additives in rats exposed by long-term inhalation. Int Arch Occup Environ Health 2001;74(2):109–18.

32. Siew SS, Kauppinen T, Kyyronen P, et al. Occupational exposure to wood dust and formaldehyde and risk of nasal, nasopharyngeal, and lung cancer among Finnish men. Cancer Manag Res 2012;4:223–32.

33. McKay SP, Gregoire L, Lonardo F, et al. Human papillomavirus (HPV) transcripts in malignant inverted papilloma are from integrated HPV DNA. Laryngoscope 2005;115(8):1428–31.

34. Frierson HF Jr, Mills SE, Fechner RE, et al. Sinonasal undifferentiated carcinoma. An aggressive neoplasm derived from schneiderian epithelium and distinct from olfactory neuroblastoma. Am J Surg Pathol 1986;10(11):771–9.

35. Chambers KJ, Lehmann AE, Remenschneider A, et al. Incidence and survival patterns of sinonasal undifferentiated carcinoma in the United States. J Neurol Surg B Skull Base 2015;76(2):94–100.

36. Lin EM, Sparano A, Spalding A, et al. Sinonasal undifferentiated carcinoma: a 13-year experience at a single institution. Skull Base 2010;20(2):61–7.

37. Xu CC, Dziegielewski PT, McGaw WT, et al. Sinonasal undifferentiated carcinoma (SNUC): the Alberta experience and literature review. J Otolaryngol Head Neck Surg 2013;42:2.

38. Reiersen DA, Pahilan ME, Devaiah AK. Meta-analysis of treatment outcomes for sinonasal undifferentiated carcinoma. Otolaryngol Head Neck Surg 2012;147(1): 7–14.

39. Ibrahim NB, Briggs JC, Corbishley CM. Extrapulmonary oat cell carcinoma. Cancer 1984;54(8):1645–61.

40. Krishnamurthy A, Ravi P, Vijayalakshmi R, et al. Small cell neuroendocrine carcinoma of the paranasal sinus. Natl J Maxillofac Surg 2013;4(1):111–3.

41. Babin E, Rouleau V, Vedrine PO, et al. Small cell neuroendocrine carcinoma of the nasal cavity and paranasal sinuses. J Laryngol Otol 2006;120(4):289–97.

42. Han G, Wang Z, Guo X, et al. Extrapulmonary small cell neuroendocrine carcinoma of the paranasal sinuses: a case report and review of the literature. J Oral Maxillofac Surg 2012;70(10):2347–51.

43. Svane-Knudsen V, Jorgensen KE, Hansen O, et al. Cancer of the nasal cavity and paranasal sinuses: a series of 115 patients. Rhinology 1998;36(1):12–4.

44. Bak M, Wein RO. Esthesioneuroblastoma: a contemporary review of diagnosis and management. Hematol Oncol Clin North Am 2012;26(6):1185–207.

45. Cohen ZR, Marmor E, Fuller GN, et al. Misdiagnosis of olfactory neuroblastoma. Neurosurg Focus 2002;12(5):e3.

46. Tufano RP, Mokadam NA, Montone KT, et al. Malignant tumors of the nose and paranasal sinuses: hospital of the University of Pennsylvania experience 1990-1997. Am J Rhinol 1999;13(2):117–23.

47. Devaiah AK, Andreoli MT. Treatment of esthesioneuroblastoma: a 16-year meta-analysis of 361 patients. Laryngoscope 2009;119(7):1412–6.

48. Tajudeen BA, Arshi A, Suh JD, et al. Esthesioneuroblastoma: an update on the UCLA experience, 2002-2013. J Neurol Surg B Skull Base 2015;76(1):43–9.

49. de Gabory L, Abdulkhaleq HM, Darrouzet V, et al. Long-term results of 28 esthesioneuroblastomas managed over 35 years. Head Neck 2011;33(1):82–6.

50. McLean JN, Nunley SR, Klass C, et al. Combined modality therapy of esthesioneuroblastoma. Otolaryngol Head Neck Surg 2007;136(6):998–1002.

51. Kim HJ, Kim CH, Lee BJ, et al. Surgical treatment versus concurrent chemoradiotherapy as an initial treatment modality in advanced olfactory neuroblastoma. Auris Nasus Larynx 2007;34(4):493–8.
52. Levine PA, Gallagher R, Cantrell RW. Esthesioneuroblastoma: reflections of a 21-year experience. Laryngoscope 1999;109(10):1539–43.
53. Dulguerov P, Allal AS, Calcaterra TC. Esthesioneuroblastoma: a meta-analysis and review. Lancet Oncol 2001;2(11):683–90.
54. Lu NN, Li YX, Wang WH, et al. Clinical behavior and treatment outcome of primary nasal diffuse large B-cell lymphoma. Cancer 2012;118(6):1593–8.
55. Kanumuri VV, Khan MN, Vazquez A, et al. Diffuse large B-cell lymphoma of the sinonasal tract: analysis of survival in 852 cases. Am J Otolaryngol 2014;35(2): 154–8.
56. Hatta C, Ogasawara H, Okita J, et al. Non-Hodgkin's malignant lymphoma of the sinonasal tract–treatment outcome for 53 patients according to REAL classification. Auris Nasus Larynx 2001;28(1):55–60.
57. Draf W. Endonasal frontal sinus drainage type I-III according to Draf. In: Kountakis S, Senior B, Draf W, editors. The frontal sinus. Germany: Springer; 2005. p. 220–32.
58. Sieśkiewicz A, Lyson T, Piszczatowski B, et al. Endoscopic treatment of adversely located osteomas of the frontal sinus. Ann Otol Rhinol Laryngol 2012;121(8): 503–9.
59. Ledderose GJ, Betz CS, Stelter K, et al. Surgical management of osteomas of the frontal recess and sinus: extending the limits of the endoscopic approach. Eur Arch Otorhinolaryngol 2010;268(4):525–32.
60. Seiberling K, Floreani S, Robinson S, et al. Endoscopic management of frontal sinus osteomas revisited. Am J Rhinol Allergy 2009;23:331–6.
61. Schaitkin B. Endoscopic approach to the frontal sinus. In: Myers E, editor. Operative otolaryngology: head and neck surgery: expert consult: online, print and video, 2-volume set. Philadelphia: Elsevier Health Sciences; 2008. p. 121–6.
62. Naidoo Y, Wormald P-J. Frontal sinus surgery. In: Johnson J, Rosen C, editors. Head and neck surgery: otolaryngology. Lippincott Williams & Wilkins, US; 2013. p. 675–87.
63. Weber R, Draf W, Kratzsch B, et al. Modern Concepts of Frontal Sinus Surgery. Laryngoscope 2001;111(1):137–46.
64. Thong J, Chatterjee D, Hwang S. Endoscopic modified Lothrop approach for the excision of bilateral frontal sinus tumors. Ear Nose Throat J 2014;93(3):116–9.
65. Conger BT, Riley K, Woodworth BA. The Draf III mucosal grafting technique: a prospective study. Otolaryngol Head Neck Surg 2012;146(4):664–8.
66. Selva D, White VA, O'Connell JX, et al. Primary bone tumors of the orbit. Surv Ophthalmol 2004;49(3):328–42.
67. Gibson T, Walker FM. Large osteoma of the frontal sinus; a method of removal to minimize scarring and prevent deformity. Br J Plast Surg 1951;4(3):210–7.

Open Frontal Sinus Surgery
A Lost Art

William Lawson, MD, DDS*, Yan Ho, MD

KEYWORDS

- Open approach frontal sinus • Open frontal sinusotomy • Frontoethmoidectomy
- Osteoplastic flap • Trephination

KEY POINTS

- External frontal sinus surgery primarily involves 3 different surgical procedures: frontal trephination, external frontoethmoidectomy, and osteoplastic flap.
- Preserve or improve drainage from frontal sinus by maintaining patency of the frontal drainage pathway.
- Attain long-term success for obliteration or cranialization of the sinuses, if necessary.
- Achieve an aesthetic outcome by preserving the natural contour of the forehead, nose, and orbit as well as minimizing scar formation.

PREOPERATIVE PLANNING AND PREPARATION

A thorough history and physical examination of patients is an important step in preoperative planning. The history should include chronicity, frequency, severity, and progression of symptoms. Because frontal sinusitis often occurs in the setting of acute or chronic rhinosinusitis, and may be exacerbated by allergic rhinitis or other types of rhinitis, it is prudent to inquire about any history of allergies or medications, including antibiotics, steroids, or immunomodulators. Any previous medical treatments or surgeries should be explored, and any history of trauma should be discussed. Attention should be paid to signs of possible orbital or intracranial complications, including changes in vision, neck stiffness, and headache.

On physical examination, vitals and a basic head and neck examination is expected. Attention should be directed toward any signs of ocular or intracranial involvement including cellulitis, erosion of the frontal bone (Pott puffy tumor), previous surgery, or scars. For example, decrease in visual acuity, gaze palsies, meningeal signs, changes in cranial nerve function, or changes in mental status should raise suspicion

Disclosures: None.
Department of Otolaryngology - Head and Neck Surgery, Icahn School of Medicine at Mount Sinai, One Gustave L Levy Place, Box 1189, New York, NY 10029-6574, USA
* Corresponding author.
E-mail address: Willam.lawson@mountsinai.org

Otolaryngol Clin N Am 49 (2016) 1067–1089
http://dx.doi.org/10.1016/j.otc.2016.03.027
0030-6665/16/$ – see front matter © 2016 Elsevier Inc. All rights reserved.

for complications of frontal sinus disease. Nasal endoscopy is a helpful and, arguably, required part of the physical examination. This procedure is important for possibly obtaining cultures and looking for anatomic abnormalities or previous surgery, signs of polyps, or other masses.

Laboratory testing is certainly a helpful adjunct to the evaluation of patients. A complete blood count can reveal an abnormal white count or a left shift, and a basic metabolic panel can detect electrolyte abnormalities or dehydration. If patients are likely to need an operative procedure, a coagulation panel (prothrombin time, partial thromboplastin time) may be helpful. Allergy testing or immunologic tests may be helpful in the outpatient setting to detect allergens or immunodeficiencies but is unlikely to be helpful in the acute setting. Nasal cultures, when collected successfully, are important for guiding antibiotic therapy; cerebrospinal fluid (CSF) or blood cultures are certainly recommended if patients show signs of altered mental status or sepsis.

A variety of radiographic tools are available. The most basic tool is a radiograph of the sinuses. This radiograph may show the general anatomy of the sinuses. If an osteoplastic flap is planned, the 6-foot occipitofrontal (Caldwell) view may be useful. At present, most physicians would order a computed tomography (CT) of the paranasal sinuses as the first step. This modality provides the most information about bony anatomy, opacification, or air-fluid levels in each of the sinuses. If obtained with contrast, it can also detect abscesses or fluid collections. MRI will provide soft tissue information but is usually not the first modality to be obtained unless there is a contraindication to CT scan. Both CT and MRI may also be accessed for surgical navigation.

PATIENT POSITIONING

For any external approach to the frontal sinus, whether or not endoscopic technique is also anticipated, patients should be placed in the supine position. Turning 90° to 180° can facilitate surgical navigation or the coronal approach. In some cases, if the neurosurgical team is involved or if surgical navigation headset interferes with the surgical approach, the patients' head may be secured with a Mayfield skull clamp, which can also be registered to image guidance technologies.

PROCEDURAL APPROACH

Before the surgical procedure, the surgeon must optimize the operative conditions to minimize complications.

When approaching the frontal sinus externally, eye protection is essential. This protection can be done via a tarsorrhaphy, corneal shield, or taping the eyes closed with adhesive tape.

Decongestion of the nasal mucosa can help facilitate the visualization and opening of the frontal sinus outflow tract. If the endoscopic approach is also anticipated, decongestion of the nose with oxymetazoline or epinephrine can help with visualization and hemostasis.

Local anesthetic can be used in combination with epinephrine along the incision line and along the dissection plane to improve hemostasis and for patient comfort, particularly if the nature of the patients' situation permits or requires that procedure be performed without general anesthesia.

If preferred, surgical navigation may be used in conjunction with these procedures, although it is not required.

EXTERNAL FRONTAL SINUS SURGERY
Introduction

Technological advances have made the endonasal approach the dominant method of frontal sinus surgery, eclipsing the more aggressive external procedures. However, they all have a specific role in contemporary rhinologic surgery. The 6 procedures described in this article are linked with endonasal surgery and use endoscopes adjunctively. Clinical experience over a century has refined them with regard to indications, clinical efficacy, and cosmetic result. Increasing uses of frontal trephination has expanded the role of endoscopic frontal sinusotomy in the management of chronic inflammatory disease and is essential for control of acute suppuration. The external frontoethmoidectomy is essentially a transorbital approach that can be used selectively for frontal, ethmoid, skull base, or orbital disease. It is indispensable for control of orbital infections and hemorrhages. In select cases it can be used in place of an osteoplastic flap. The frontal osteoplastic flap is the most invasive procedure and is reserved for inflammatory disease that has failed intranasal and external procedures; it is also used for disease processes of the frontal sinus that cannot be accessed or completely removed transnasally. It must be remembered that although chronic sinusitis is the most common condition treated, the frontal sinus is the host of diverse lesions, including mucoceles, allergic fungal sinusitis, osteomyelitis, as well as neoplasms, pneumatoceles, encephaloceles, and traumatic injuries. Accordingly, in undertaking the treatment of frontal sinus disease, one must make concessions: first that one procedure or approach cannot treat all diseases and second that there is a subset of patients who defy long-term cure.

Even the most experienced endoscopic surgeons retain them in the surgical armamentarium for the complete treatment of frontal sinus disease. As an example, Hahn and colleagues[1] reported that of 717 procedures in 683 patients done for inflammatory disease, in the period from 2004 to 2008, at the University of Pennsylvania, 5.3% underwent external procedures, consisting of 24 osteoplastic flaps and 14 trephines. These procedures were most often used when the frontal recess was stenosed by osteoneogenesis from previous surgeries.

FRONTAL TREPHINE
Introduction

The frontal trephine had its origin as a direct method of evacuating purulent material from an acutely infected sinus or one with chronic infection and osteomyelitis. With the shift from external to endoscopic surgery for the management of frontal sinus disease, it became apparent that the purely transnasal approach could not completely address the complex anatomy and diverse pathology of the frontal sinus. The frontal trephine now serves as a secondary tool, expanding the scope and treatment of cases previously requiring an osteoplastic flap.[2]

Its present reincarnation is called mini-trephination and uses endoscopic visualization and instruments. Even the most experienced endoscopic surgeons recognize its value in managing difficult primary and revision cases. Seiberling and colleagues[3] reported that 188 trephinations were made during 80 modified Lothrop procedures and 108 frontal sinusotomies over an 8-year period at the University of Adelaide, South Australia with a complication rate of 5.4%. In their series, indications included extensive polyposis, fungal sinusitis, aberrant ethmoid air cells, or a stenosed outflow tract. The combined use has been referred to as the above-and-below approach.

History

In 1884, Ogston[4] published the first external approach to the frontal sinus in which he performed a trephine through the anterior table and created a drainage pathway into the nose through the anterior ethmoid air cells. Luc[5] performed a similar procedure in 1896. The procedure is reminiscent of what is done today for an acute frontal sinusitis whereby the purulent secretions are evacuated externally and an endonasal drainage pathway is created.[6]

Indications

- Acute frontal sinusitis: Acute sinusitis with an air-fluid level within the frontal sinus is a major indication, especially when there is radiographic evidence of dural enhancement or suggestion of an epidural abscess (**Fig. 1**). Intense nasal congestion may preclude safe intranasal drainage and a patent sinusotomy by endoscopic surgery alone.[7]
- Chronic frontal sinusitis or frontal osteomyelitis: Chronic sinusitis with an air-fluid level that has not responded to medical therapy and endoscopic surgery is especially difficult to access; trephination is helpful if orbital or intracranial (**Fig. 2**).
- Biopsy of frontal sinus lesions: Trephination provides a direct route for biopsy of lesions within the frontal sinus that are not accessible with an endonasal approach.
- Repair of frontal sinus fractures: Depressed fractures of the anterior table can be elevated through a trephine with a curved clamp or sound, with placement of a balloon catheter inside the sinus if the fracture segments are unstable (**Fig. 3**).
- Expanding the scope of endoscopic frontal sinusotomy:
  ○ It facilitates the opening and removal of agger nasi cells and type III and IV frontal cells that extend into the frontal sinus[8,9] (**Fig. 4**).
  ○ It facilitates the drainage of an infected interseptal frontal air cell.
  ○ It can be used for frontal sinus septectomy to drain a sinus with an obstructive outflow tract into the normal unobstructed side.
  ○ With a developmentally narrow outflow tract or one that is contracted by osteoneogenesis or fibrosis, placement of contrast materials and retrograde cannulation into the nose can be performed with a malleable probe, permitting safe creation of a Draf IIb procedure.

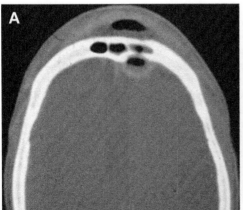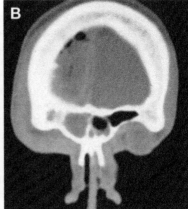

Fig. 1. Axial (*A*) and coronal (*B*) CT with subgaleal and epidural abscess secondary to frontal sinusitis.

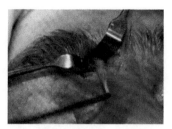

Fig. 2. Frontal sinus with dense secretions aspirated through trephine.

- It can provide access laterally to facilitate endoscopic frontal sinusotomy drainage of a sequestered lateral supraorbital ethmoid or septated frontal sinus mucocele.
- Other subsidiary uses are to facilitate management of nasal polyposis, for postoperative irrigation after frontal sinusotomy (**Fig. 5**), and to facilitate stent placement (**Fig. 6**).

Technique

In the preantibiotic era, opening into a chronically infected frontal sinus was through the floor of the sinus, not only because it was the thinnest wall but it also lacked diploe through which infection could spread. Over the years, this technique has been preserved for the indications listed previously. It can be safely performed through a 1.5-cm opening at, or slightly anterior, to the medial aspect of the eyebrow. An incision is made down to the periosteum, and hemostasis is achieved with bipolar cautery. After the periosteum is incised and elevated, an opening is made with a 4-mm cutting burr at the junction of the medial and superior orbital walls, at the anterior border of the supraorbital ridge. The bone is thinned to a blue lining through which the sinus can be visualized and safely opened; enlargement with Kerrison-type punches is performed depending on the size of the opening required. After the sinus contents are aspirated and cultured, an endoscope can be inserted to visualize all the recesses of the sinus. If a trephine is performed for infection, a thin rubber catheter can be inserted for drainage and irrigation. The incision is then closed with 4-0 deep absorbable sutures and a continuous 6-0 nylon or polypropylene suture for the skin.

Complications

Careful evaluation of a multi-planar CT scan is essential to evaluate the depth of the sinus and location of the intersinus septum to avoid misplacement of the trephine

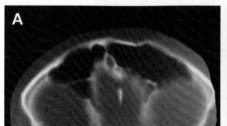
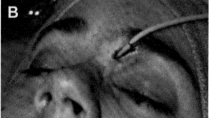

Fig. 3. (*A*) Anterior table fracture reduced through trephine and (*B*) stabilized with balloon catheter.

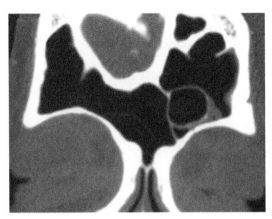

Fig. 4. Type IV cell in left frontal sinus.

opening. The position of the incision should not be within the eyebrow as an area of alopecia may develop. Careful layered closure should produce an imperceptible incision line. The trephine should be placed at the medial-most portion of the supra-orbital ridge, as placement further laterally may injure the supratrochlear or supraorbital nerves with regional paresthesias. Misplacement laterally can also cause injury to the trochlea with diplopia developing from disturbance of the superior oblique muscle (**Fig. 7**).

EXTERNAL FRONTOETHMOIDECTOMY
Introduction

The keystone to the management of inflammatory frontal sinus disease is restoration of its outflow tract. Technological advances in instrumentation, imaging, and navigational devices have led endonasal endoscopic surgery to be the preferred method to accomplish this. Nevertheless, frontal sinus anatomy, postoperative healing, and the

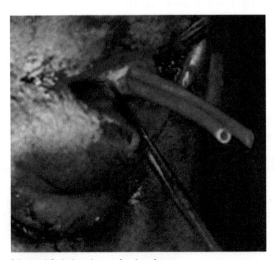

Fig. 5. Frontal trephine with irrigating tube in place.

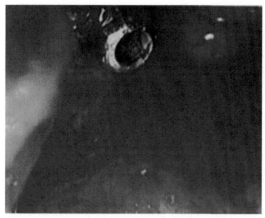

Fig. 6. Polymeric silicone tube placement through trephine after complete endoscopic sinusotomy.

type and extent of disease do not permit an endoscopic technique universally. The role of external surgery has been shifted to be an adjunct to endonasal procedures because of the limitations cited earlier. Moreover, it is the principal method of addressing the orbital and intracranial complications of sinus disease and may serve as an alternative to osteoplastic flap for the management of tumors, mucoceles, and fungal sinusitis.

The term *external frontoethmoidectomy* is being used generically for the operative management of orbital, skull base, ethmoid, and frontal disease, selectively or collectively, through a transfacial approach. In all applications, it is necessary to know the precise anatomy of the medial orbit and its relationship to the adjacent paranasal sinuses. The key structures to be recognized are the medial canthal ligament, the lacrimal sac and fossa, the ethmoidal blood vessels, and the trochlea. Frontal sinusotomy, ethmoidectomy, and orbitotomy can be performed without disruption of the nasofrontal duct, depending on the pathology.

History

Jansen[10] in 1902, and Ritter[11] in 1906, reported a transorbital approach to the frontal sinus by removing the ethmoid sinuses and creating a common cavity into the nasal cavity. In 1908, Knapp essentially described the external frontoethmoidectomy in its present form.[12] An excision under the eyebrow was carried to the lateral side of the nose between the mid dorsum and medial canthus. The periosteum was elevated

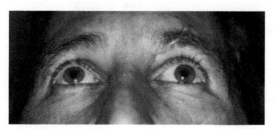

Fig. 7. Intraeyebrow incision injuring left trochlea causing superior oblique muscle dysfunction.

and the lacrimal sac was displaced, permitting removal of the floor of the frontal sinus and the ethmoid labyrinth, with placement of a drainage tube into the nose. A study of 100 skulls demonstrated the anatomy of the trochlea and that by re-apposition of the periosteum its normal position could be maintained without the development of diplopia. In 1921, Lynch[13] reported his results with 15 operations in the United States and Howarth[14] with more than 200 cases in England. Paradoxically, Lynch gained eponymic fame for devising the procedure, and the classic contribution of Knapp is generally overlooked. Lynch removed the floor of the frontal sinus, stripped all the mucosa, and drained the frontal sinuses. Howarth removed the entire floor of the frontal sinus, retained the mucosa, and performed a complete ethmoidectomy. Both surgeons used rubber tube drainage into the nose.[6]

Indications

1. Chronic frontal sinusitis: The management of chronic frontal sinusitis has undergone a massive paradigm shift from open to endonasal surgery. In addition to technological advances and better understanding of the pathophysiology, new procedures have been devised to enlarge the frontal sinus outflow tract to compensate for postoperative narrowing. These procedures have been notably the work of Draf[15] and include unilateral outflow enlargement and the resurrection of the Lothrop procedure as a purely endonasal method to conjoin both sinus outflow tracts into a common opening. In a small number of cases, the anatomy of the frontal sinus (especially the anteroposterior width) may limit endoscopic instrumentation. The external approach with stenting may eliminate or precede the use of an osteoplastic flap. With a small frontal sinus, it is possible to remove all the chronically diseased mucosa and obliterate the cavity. It provides wider access to mucoceles, often eliminating an osteoplastic flap.
2. Drainage of orbital abscesses: Subperiosteal and intraconal suppurative disease can be rapidly and directly drained. Intraorbital pressure can be reduced as needed by incising the periorbita and removal of the bone of the medial orbital wall to increase orbital volume. Disease in the ethmoid sinus, which is the usual cause of this complication, can also be treated at this time (**Fig. 8**).
3. Drainage of orbital hematomas: This procedure is essential for the management of orbital bleeding secondary to facial trauma or iatrogenic entry into the orbit. It provides access for the evacuation of the hematoma, controls the source of bleeding, and achieves orbital decompression by the removal of the medial orbital wall and drainage of blood into the nasal cavity through the ethmoid complex (**Fig. 9**).
4. Orbital decompression of endocrine exophthalmos: A variety of approaches, including the endonasal, transantral, and conjunctival, are widely used for orbital decompression of endocrine exophthalmos. The external approach is rarely used

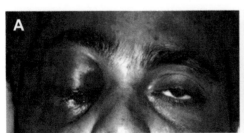
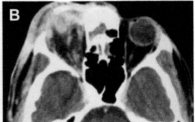

Fig. 8. (*A*) Orbital abscesses can be drained via a frontoethmoidectomy incision. (*B*) Axial CT showing orbital abscess.

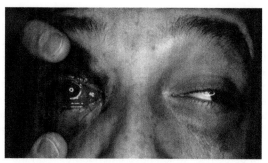

Fig. 9. Iatrogenic orbital hematoma producing extreme proptosis, chemosis, and ophthalmoplegia.

for this purpose but still has a role with unilateral disease whereby the floor of the orbit must be left intact to prevent downward displacement of the eye and the development of diplopia. In the external approach, the entire medial orbital ball can be removed with direct visualization and protection of key anatomic structures, such as the ethmoidal blood vessels, lacrimal sac, and floor of the anterior cranial fossa. A lateral approach (Kronlein) can be used adjunctively for additional orbital decompression.

5. Repair of frontal encephaloceles and CSF leaks: Through this approach, the floor of the frontal sinus can be removed, providing direct access to the posterior wall of the frontal sinus for the repair of encephaloceles and closure of CSF leaks.
6. Removal of inverted papilloma: An established cause of failure in the resection of primary and recurrent inverted papillomas is extension into the nasofrontal duct and frontal sinus **(Fig. 10)**. These tumors can be more completely removed with

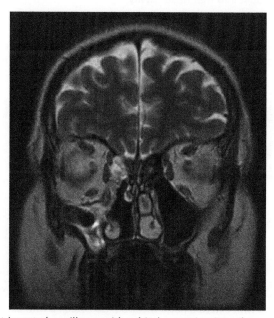

Fig. 10. Recurrent inverted papilloma with orbital extension into the medial rectus.

an open technique, along with the underlying bone, which is often involved by the tumor. For tumors having orbital extension through the lamina papyracea, the eye can be safely retracted, the lacrimal sac mobilized and retracted, and the surrounding ethmoid labyrinth exenterated.[16] It may save as a bridging procedure between endoscopic removal and the osteoplastic flap.

7. Removal of osteomas: A system of grading frontal osteomas was devised by Chiu and colleagues,[17] in 2005, who recommended that an external approach be used for lesions lateral to the sagittal plane through the lamina papyracea, those with a base of attachment anteriorly or superiorly in the frontal sinus, and those that fill the frontal sinus. A transorbital approach may be helpful to remove large frontoethmoidal osteomas, which have extended through the lamina papyracea into the orbit, fill a large part of the frontal sinus, and are attached to the skull base. The external approach permits retraction and protection of the globe and resection of any extension into the frontal sinus or adjacent skull base with repair of any dural exposures or defects (**Fig. 11**).

8. Removal of tumors: It provides for wider access through the floor of the frontal sinus for biopsy or removal of lesions of the superior and lateral recesses of the sinuses.

9. Decompression of allergic fungal sinusitis and mucoceles of the frontal sinus and orbit: Frontoethmoidectomy can be performed to remove the tenacious mucoid secretions (**Fig. 12**) and debris of allergic fungal sinusitis and to marsupialize and reduce the volume of associated mucoceles extending into the orbit and intracranially, preliminarily to definitive surgery by an osteoplastic flap. (**Fig. 13**)

10. To bypass an obstructed ethmoid labyrinth: With naso-orbito-ethmoid fractures, the frontal outflow may be totally obliterated and a new entry point into the nose is necessary. Similarly, traumatic dehiscence of the lamina papyracea may cause orbital fat to herniate into the middle meatus and obstruct the frontal outflow tract. With the transfacial approach, frontal sinus drainage is restored by creating and stenting a neoduct into that nasal cavity.

Technique

After the induction of general anesthesia, a tarsorrhaphy suture is placed. An incision is made starting beneath the medial aspect of the eyebrow, passing midway between

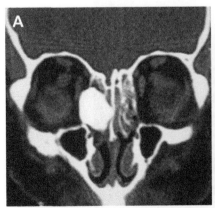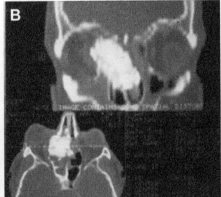

Fig. 11. (*A*) Osteoma with extension into the orbit. (*B*) Osteoma with extensive attachment to the skull base.

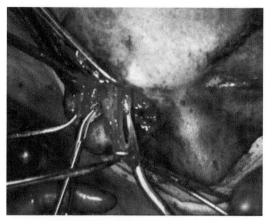

Fig. 12. Allergic fungal sinusitis with dense mucoid secretions.

the nasal dorsum and the medial canthus to a point just below the medial canthus. Dissection is carried through the soft tissues to the periosteum of the frontal process of the maxilla. Hemostasis of the angular blood vessels is achieved with bipolar cautery.

The periosteum is then incised and elevated onto the medial orbital wall. The two limbs of the medial canthal ligament are detached from the anterior and posterior crests of the lachrymal fossa. The ligament is then tagged with a suture, which is also used for retraction (**Fig. 14**). The lacrimal sac is displaced from its fossa and carefully retracted with a narrow orbital ribbon retractor for wider access to the medial orbital wall. The frontoethmoidal suture is exposed by dissection superiorly, and the anterior ethmoid artery is identified in the suture line and controlled with bipolar cautery. Its position is approximately 1.5 cm deep to the top of the lacrimal fossa, and the posterior ethmoid artery is approximately 1.0 cm behind it (**Fig. 15**). The posterior ethmoid artery is not routinely cauterized because of its proximity to the optic nerve and its role as a posterior landmark. The vessels can be clearly identified leaving the bone, with visualization enhanced by the use of endoscopes. The frontoethmoidal suture line and ethmoidal vessels are important landmarks as they correspond to the floor of the anterior cranial fossa and, hence, are the superior limits of dissection.

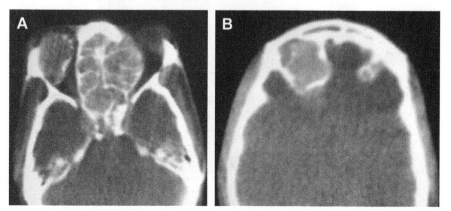

Fig. 13. Axial CT showing (*A*) orbital and (*B*) intracranial extension of mucocele.

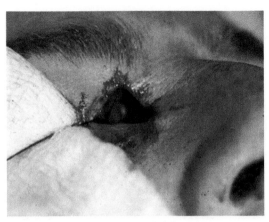

Fig. 14. Detachment and tagging of medial canthal ligament.

The bone of the lacrimal fossa and the lamina papyracea are perforated, and the labyrinth is exenterated completely through the orbit and also endoscopically, remaining lateral to the middle turbinate. If necessary for orbital decompression, bone can be removed inferiorly to the level of the infraorbital canal. Removal of the bone directly above the lacrimal fossa with a Kerrison rongeur will lead into the frontal sinus. Bone can be selectively removed from the floor of the frontal sinus depending on the necessity for access to the lateral recess. The frontal sinus is then inspected with endoscopes. Additional bone is removed along the frontonasal outflow tract to create the maximum opening into the nose. A resection of a portion of the middle

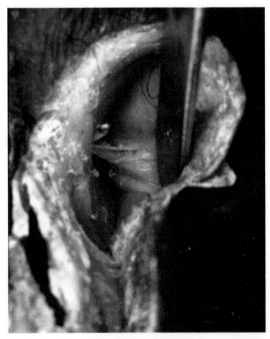

Fig. 15. Key landmarks in the intraorbital approach: lacrimal sac and anterior ethmoid artery.

turbinate may be required, and the neoduct is then stented with a polymeric silicon tube or a sheet of rolled polymeric silicon, which is then anchored to the nasal septum with a 3-0 nylon suture. The periosteum is now meticulously coapted with 4-0 poly-glactin 910 sutures, as this repositions the trochlea and the medial canthal ligament to its original position. The subcutaneous tissues are closed with 4-0 chromic catgut sutures and the skin closed with a continuous 6-0 nylon suture. A strip of antibiotic petrolatum dressing gauze is placed over the incision.

Complications

The greatest limitation of the external frontoethmoidectomy in treating chronic frontal sinus disease is closure of the nasofrontal duct by fibrosis and osteoneogenesis. This closure results in persistent and recurrent infection and secondary mucocele forma-tion. Accordingly, the success rate of the procedure decreases with time. This circum-stance has led to more aggressive endonasal sinusotomies to increase the patency rates.

To maintain nasofrontal duct patency outflow, a variety of methods of stenting and resurfacing of this area have been devised. Various metallic and synthetic substances have been used for stenting; however, patency has not been found to be related to the biocompatibility of the alloplastic material. The interval to closure of the neoduct has been found to be from months to several years until stenosis occurs. Resurfacing of the surgical neoduct has been attempted by the applications of grafts and the rotation of local mucosal flaps. Free mucosal and skin grafts have been used and found to be ineffective. A variety of medially and laterally based mucosal flaps have been devised with varying success. In 1998, Dedo and colleagues[18] reported a failed patency rate of 3% in 36 cases that were followed for a mean of 6 years.

Long-term stenting for chronic disease has been used with both endoscopic and external surgeries. Indications for its placement include neo-ostium openings less than 5 mm, extensive polyposis, circumferential demucosalization, flail middle turbi-nate, and fracture of the outflow tract. Amble and colleagues[19] reported stenting 164 cases for inflammatory disease, or mucoceles, with an 18% revision rate after a mean follow-up of 47 months, with no major complications and 3.2% minor complica-tions. Benoit and Duncavage[20] used stents in combined endoscopic and external frontal sinusotomies in 40 patients (total of 62 procedures) and achieved a 72% patency rate, with a 12-month follow-up period.[20] In 2001, Rains[21] describes the use of a self-retaining silicone tube for frontal sinus disease in 67 patients.

A variety of intraoperative complications due to injury to adjacent anatomic struc-tures are possible. Overall, hematomas can result from incomplete control of the ethmoidal blood vessels. Hemostasis is effectively achieved by bipolar electrocau-tery, whereas clip ligation is less secure as the clips may become dislodged. Vision loss is a potential complication from direct injury to the optic nerve from dissection too far posteriorly into the orbit. Identifying and leaving the posterior ethmoid artery intact protects the area of the optic foramen. Injury to the lacrimal sac may result in epiphora or dacryocystitis. The lacrimal sac should be dissected totally free from its fossa and gently retracted; it is not to be compressed directly with orbital retrac-tors. Surgical dissection along the roof of the orbit may result in damage to the trochlea and result in diplopia from superior oblique imbalance. Careful elevation of the periorbita and meticulous suturing of the periosteal layer will avoid this. Failure to reattach the medial canthal ligament can result in pseudohypertelorism. Tagging the ligament after it is detached with a suture and reattaching it to the periosteum of the frontomaxillary process with a permanent suture eliminates this. Entry into the anterior cranial fossa and development of a CSF leak can be prevented by identifying the frontoethmoidal suture line with the ethmoidal vessels running through it and never going superior to this suture line. Entry into the frontal sinus should always be on a vertical path directly above the lacrimal fossa. The possibility of unsatisfactory scar formation can be limited by a meticulous layered closure using 6-0 nylon for the skin. The incision should be placed midway between the nasal dorsum and the medial canthus, as an incision too close to the medial canthus will result in the formation of a web.

FRONTAL OSTEOPLASTIC FLAP
History

In 1894, the first reports of entry into the frontal sinus by creating a hinged osteoperiosteal flap were made by Schonborn in Europe.[22] In 1898, Brieger reported that the bone flap was temporarily removed during the procedure.[23] The application of fat to obliterate the sinus was made by Marx[24] in 1910 and was introduced by Bergara and Itoiz[26] and Tato and colleagues[27] in the 1930s and 1940s in South America. The publications of Goodale and Montgomery[28] in the 1950s popularized this procedure in the United States. The collective experience of 250 cases reported by Hardy and Montgomery,[25] in 1976, firmly established its role in the management of frontal sinus disease.

Frontal Osteoplastic Flap Principles

1. The osteoplastic flap should be performed after the other paranasal sinuses have been treated and are free of disease.
2. The osteoplastic flap should not be performed in the presence of acute infection, as it places the bone flap at risk and may lead to necrosis of the fat graft and produce a wound infection.
3. A sufficient amount of viable bone must be present (estimated at more than 50%) for fat graft survival; if insufficient bone is present, cranialization should be considered.
4. It is essential to remove all the mucosa from the surgical cavity to prevent secondary mucocele formation.
   a. The nasofrontal ducts should be stripped of their lining and plugged with another autogenous tissue, not relying solely on the fat for closure as it may retract and permit reepithelialization.
   b. Mucosa should be removed from all of the crevices. The bone should be burred to remove epithelial remnants present along the diploic veins of Breschet as well as to decorticate the anterior and posterior tables to promote neovascularization of the fat graft.
   c. Supraorbital ethmoids must be unroofed and all the mucosa removed. This may be technically difficult or even impossible. Weber and colleagues had to retract the dura in 6 cases to facilitate clearing of supraorbital ethmoid cells.[29]
   d. The patients with mucoceles eroding bone and in contact with the periorbita or dura are almost impossible to totally de-epithelialize and predispose patients to recurrence of the mucocele.
5. The implantation material of choice is abdominal fat as it has resulted in less complications in filling the sinus cavity than other autologous materials. The use of alloplastic materials carries a high rate of complications and often results in re-exploration and revision.
6. Minimizing bone loss and careful preservation and approximation of the periosteum reduces the occurrence of forehead irregularities.

Indications

In virtually all studies, the frontal osteoplastic flap is used selectively in patients with chronic sinusitis, osteomas, mucoceles, and fractures. Less common indications include osteomyelitis, infection of implant material, CSF leaks, and pneumatoceles.

Chronic sinusitis

Techniques to enlarge the frontal sinus outflow tract to compensate for postsurgical narrowing coupled with navigational devices have dominated the management of chronic sinusitis. However, instances in which it is not possible to maintain a patent opening will lead to an external approach for disease control.[1,3] Also, massive recurrent polyposis, allergic fungal sinusitis, and foci of osteomyelitis may dictate a direct approach (**Fig. 16**).

Mucoceles

Presently, most frontal and frontoethmoidal mucoceles are treated endoscopically. Marsupialization of the mucocele into the nasal cavity is highly effective and desirable with those adherent to the periorbita or dura whereby total removal of the wall is difficult and recurrence is common. Nevertheless, in all series there are a small number of mucoceles that require an external approach. These mucoceles are generally are recurrent and are sequestered laterally by scarring or osteoneogenesis or in constricted frontal sinuses where an adequate opening into the nose cannot be obtained[30] (**Fig. 17**).

Osteomas and other tumors

Although osteomas are the most prevalent neoplasm of the frontal sinus, inverted papillomas, meningiomas, fibro-osseous lesions, and hemangiomas also occur. With osteomas, it is important to completely remove the base of the lesion as regrowth can occur years later (**Fig. 18**).

Fractures

Fractures involving the frontal outflow tract and the posterior table are considered candidates for sinus obliteration: the former because of the high incidence of secondary mucoceles and the latter because of direct exposure and/or laceration of the dura, with the development of CSF leaks and meningitis. Severely comminuted fractures with extensive fragmentation can form loculations in the sinus by fibrosis and osteogenesis, resulting in the delayed development of mucopyoceles and chronic osteomyelitis. Surgical exploration will determine if they are best obliterated by fat or cranialized.

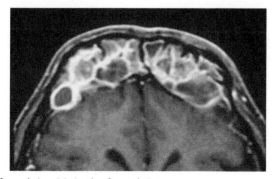

Fig. 16. Allergic fungal sinusitis in the frontal sinuses.

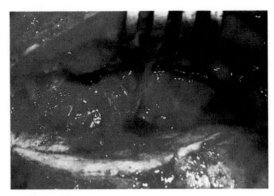

Fig. 17. Frontal sinus filled with mucus.

Correction of pneumatoceles

Hyperaeration of the frontal sinus causing extensive frontal bossing and cosmetic deformity can be corrected with the frontal osteoplastic flap with fat obliteration. The expanded anterior table can be recessed into the sinus cavity thereby recontouring the area and the nasofrontal duct closed with fascia and fat eliminating the ball valve effect causing the deformity (**Fig. 19**).

Technique

Before the procedure is performed, the creation of an accurate template demonstrating the borders of the frontal sinuses is fabricated from a 6-ft Caldwell view (posteroanterior) plain radiograph to minimize any magnification error. To confirm its accuracy, a linear measurement is made from the superolateral junction from one orbit

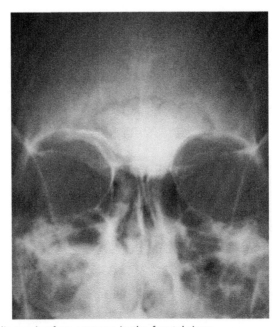

Fig. 18. Plain radiograph of an osteoma in the frontal sinus.

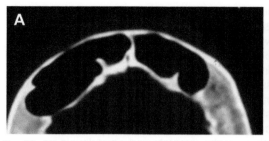
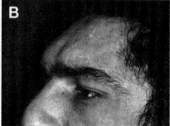

Fig. 19. (*A*) Frontal pneumatocele causing (*B*) external deformity.

to that of the opposite side; a comparable measurement should be found on the radiograph. The template is stored in an iodophor solution until it is needed for the procedure (**Fig. 20**).

The intersinus septum and the sides are scratched into the template for correct placement. The position of the incision is determined by the patients' hairline or the presence of a previous incision. This incision generally takes the form of a gull wing or coronal incision, but midforehead incisions have also been used.

A gull wing type of incision follows the eyebrow and extends down over the nasal glabella region to the opposite eyebrow. The incision may be placed above the eyebrow, within the eyebrow, or beneath the eyebrow. An incision within the eyebrow often creates areas of alopecia and a visible incision line despite beveling. An incision beneath the eyebrow passes through a thick layer of muscle and is accompanied by bleeding and requires more extensive hemostasis. The authors prefer the incision along the upper border of the eyebrow as it creates a thinner and more pliable flap. The coronal incision gives optimal camouflage and exposure, preserves the superior and supratrochlear neurovascular bundles, and provides access for the harvesting of temporalis fascia grafts. It is placed more posteriorly over the vertex of the head in patients with a receding hairline.

After the induction of general anesthesia, tarsorrhaphy sutures are placed and the face and scalp are prepped and draped. With the coronal incision, a 2- to 3-cm strip of hair is shaved behind the hairline and an incision is marked from the superior attachment of one ear across the vertex to the same area on the opposite side. The scalp should be infiltrated with 1% lidocaine and epinephrine 1:100,000 along the incision line, approximately 10 minutes before the procedure begins. This

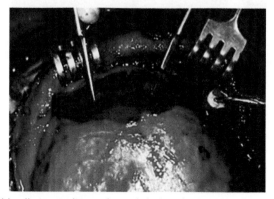

Fig. 20. A 6-ft Caldwell view radiograph used during the surgery.

infiltration markedly reduces incisional bleeding, which can be readily controlled with bipolar cautery, keeping blood loss less than 100 mL. Alternatively, scalp clips can be applied. The scalp is incised down to the pericranium, and the flap is elevated by sharp dissection in the subgaleal plane to approximately 3 cm above the supraorbital ridges. Laterally, the dissection is in the loose areolar tissue over the temporalis fascia and superficial temporal blood vessels. The flap is reflected down over the face; using blunt dissection, the supratrochlear and supraorbital nerves are identified and preserved. The template is then positioned over the lower border of the supraorbital ridges and onto the glabellar region where it is fixed in place with scalpels. The periosteum is incised along the periphery of the template and carefully elevated 2 to 3 mm along the proposed site of the osteotomy. With a unilateral flap, the pericranium is incised centrally along the line of the intersinus septum, which had been previously marked on the template. The bone is sectioned carefully with an oscillating saw to minimize bone loss. The bone cut is markedly beveled to prevent penetration of the posterior table, as in some patients the superior angle of the frontal sinus is extremely shallow, and also to compensate for a slight magnification error in constructing the template. Lateral osteotomies are made with the saw through the dense bone of the supraorbital ridges to a depth of 1 cm, which prevents fracture of the bone flap on elevation. A curved chisel is then used to sever the intersinus septum, and the bone flap is elevated carefully keeping it hinged inferiorly on the periosteum (**Fig. 21**).

The soft tissue contents of the sinus are removed from the anterior and posterior tables and from all the crevices. This procedure is followed by drilling the bony walls of the cavity with round cutting and diamond burrs. It is important at this point to have removed all the mucosal elements, stripped the nasofrontal ducts, unroofed supraorbital ethmoid cells, and removed the mucosa that extends from them along the posterior wall of the orbit (**Fig. 22**).

The burring down of the posterior table removes unseen remnants of mucosa that follow the veins of Breschet and provides a fine bleeding bed for the revascularization of the adipose/graft. The cavities are irrigated extensively with saline, and a segment of temporalis fascia is harvested and used to fill the denuded nasofrontal ducts. The

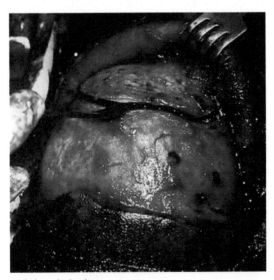

Fig. 21. Bone flap with beveled edges.

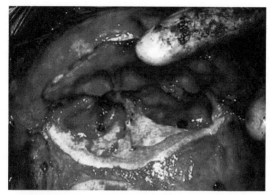

Fig. 22. Frontal sinus with all of the mucosa stripped.

fascia is then overlaid with freshly harvested adipose tissue removed from a prepared abdominal site (**Fig. 23**).

Each sinus should be completely filled with fat but not compressed when the bone flap is returned to its original position. It is stabilized by a single 28-gauge wire (or thin plates with screws), and the periosteum is meticulously approximated with 4-0 polyglactin 910 sutures. Additional hemostasis is obtained; a small Penrose drain is placed on both sides, and the scalp flap is returned to its original position.

The incision is closed with 2-0 absorbable sutures for the galeal layer and a continuous 3-0 polypropylene suture for the skin. The incision is coated with bacitracin ointment, overlaid with xeroform gauze; a light dressing of fluffed gauze is placed over the forehead. Care is taken not to apply too much compression, as this will result in upper eyelid edema. The abdominal incision also receives a layered closure with 3-0 absorbable sutures for the deep tissues, a continuous nylon or Monocryl suture for the skin, after the placement of a small Penrose drain. The wounds are redressed, and the drains are removed the following morning.

Complications

The success rate and limitations of the osteoplastic flap have to be viewed in perspective. Complications of the frontal osteoplastic flap are related to the nature of the operative procedure, the anatomy and properties of the frontal sinus itself, and the type of

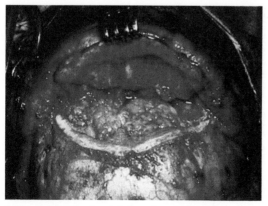

Fig. 23. Fat graft placed within the frontal sinus for obliteration.

pathology treated. Certain features of the frontal sinuses tend to defeat surgery. These features include its anatomic relationship to the adjunctive sinuses, the propensity of mucocele formation, osteoneogenesis, and its intimate relationship to the orbit and intracranial structures. Intrinsic in performing the osteoplastic flap, there are several challenges:

- The necessity of removing all the mucosa
- The potential of an orbital or intracranial complication
- The development of embossment and frontal contour abnormalities
- Changes or intolerance of the implanted material

Finally, the osteoplastic flap is the end-game procedure for patients with frontal sinus disease who have failed all medical and surgical treatment. Endoscopy has dramatically changed the treatment of frontal sinus disease, especially chronic sinusitis; but there are conditions beyond the scope of management that requires a direct approach.

The 82 osteoplastic flaps reported by Weber and colleagues represent endonasal cases performed by the most experienced surgeons who had devised many of these procedures.[19] These cases represent advanced sinus disease that has bone thinning and erosion, dural and periorbital exposure and attachments, distorted anatomy by mucoceles, and fractures that directly influence the intraoperative complication rates.[29] Consequently, the meticulous cataloging of complications accompanying these articles reflects the clinical difficulty of these cases. Their success rate of 90% confirms that frontal sinus disease cannot universally be cured by surgery and there is a small number of patients who carry the potential burden of numerous revisions on prolonged follow-up.

Intraoperative complications are principally intracranial injury, orbital fat herniation, bone flap fracture, or malposition. Postoperative complications may be grouped into cosmetic, neurologic, mucocele formation, and miscellaneous, which include fistulas and osteomyelitis (**Fig. 24**).

Operative complications include dural injury from an inaccurate template or its faulty placement. Fractured bone flaps can result from inadequate osteotomies along the supraorbital ridges or excessive thinning or attachment of an osteoma to the anterior table. Orbital injury can arise from fracture of the orbital roof on elevation of the bone flap or in an attempt to remove all the mucosa of the supraorbital ethmoid cell by burring down its borders. Surgery for chronic disease may lead to infection

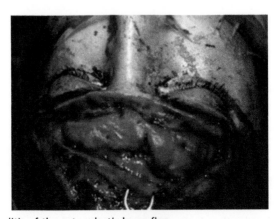

Fig. 24. Osteomyelitis of the osteoplastic bone flap.

of the operative site resulting in cellulitis, abscess, or fistula formation. Continued bleeding in the operative field may lead to the formation of a hematoma or seroma. The donor site for the abdominal fat graft may also develop a seroma, hematoma, or infection.

Postoperative complications include an unsatisfactory scar with areas of alopecia developing despite beveling of the skin incision. Frontal contour irregularities may result from areas of bone loss from the osteotomy or resorption secondary to the loss of the overlying periosteum. Specific to the frontal sinus is the development of embossment secondary to hypertrophy of the bone flap, not to be confused with flap migration from lack of adequate fixation (**Fig. 25**).

Paresthesias and anesthesia of the forehead result from an injury to the supraorbital and supratrochlear nerves, which are often permanent with the gull-wing incision, which transects the nerves; however, they are only temporary with distally placed coronal incisions. Some patients develop a chronic frontal pain syndrome regionally that may last months or even years. It has been misdiagnosed as representing recurrent disease and has lead to negative re-explorations of the sinus. Consequently, objective signs of infection (forehead swelling, local tenderness, fistula, periorbital edema) should be present before surgery is performed. Attempts to differentiate symptomatic from asymptomatic patients based on MRI findings has not been successful. The amount of residual fat remnant does not necessarily correlate with the clinical findings. The major postoperative complication of the osteoplastic flap is the occurrence of mucoceles secondary to proliferation of minute mucosal remnants or from residual epithelium from the mucoceles that have been removed, especially those contacting the dura or periorbita.

Summary

Currently, the osteoplastic flap is less often performed for chronic inflammatory disease. However, its indications are well defined in numerous publications, both as a primary and salvage procedure. Template construction has been by plain radiograph, transillumination through a trephine, and by navigational devices, all having comparable accuracy. Although it is most commonly performed with abdominal fat obliteration, in some cases obliteration is not performed and a large communication into the nasal cavity is created by modified endoscopic Lothrop procedure.

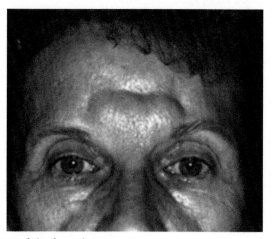

Fig. 25. Embossment of the frontal sinus.

The potential complications of the procedure are also well established and can be reduced by surgical experience.

SUMMARY

Although the 3 external procedures discussed are more than a century old, they continue to have a role in contemporary rhinologic surgery. The role of the frontal trephine is now greater because of its utility in expanding the role of endoscopic frontal sinusotomy. The role of external frontoethmoidectomy in treating chronic sinusitis has decreased because of its high incidence of stenosis. However, in highly selective cases it is performed where a neo-ostium is to be created. However, knowledge of this transfacial, transorbital approach is essential in managing orbital infections and hemorrhage and for application to select cases of the frontal, ethmoid, and skull-base lesions. Finally, the osteoplastic flap performed with fat obliteration remains the salvage procedure of failed external and endoscopic procedures and can be used as a primary procedure for laterally based frontal sinus lesions and traumatic deformities.

REFERENCES

1. Hahn S, Palmer JN, Purkey MT, et al. Indications for external frontal sinus procedures for inflammatory sinus disease. Am J Rhinol Allergy 2009;23(3):342–7.
2. Patel AB, Cain RB, Lal D. Contemporary applications of frontal sinus trephination: a systematic review of the literature. Laryngoscope 2015;125(9):2046–53.
3. Seiberling K, Jardeleza C, Wormald P. Minitrephination of the frontal sinus: indications and uses in today's era of sinus surgery. Am J Rhinol Allergy 2009; 23(2):229–31.
4. Ogston A. Trephining the frontal sinus for catarrhal diseases. Men Chron Manchester 1884;1:235.
5. Luc H. Traitement des sinuses fontales suppures chroniques par l'ouverture largesse de la paroi antérieure du sinus et le drainage par la voie nasale (méthode d'Ogston et Luc). Arch Int Laryngol 1896;9:163.
6. Lawson W. Frontal sinus. In: Blitzer A, Lawson W, Friedman WH, editors. Surgery of the paranasal sinuses. Philadelphia: WB Saunders; 1991. p. 183–217.
7. Mortimore S, Wormald P. Management of acute complicated sinusitis: a 5-year review. Otolaryngol Head Neck Surg 1999;121:639–42.
8. Maeso P, Deal RT, Kountakis SE. Combined endoscopic and minitrephination techniques in the surgical management of frontal sinus type IV cell disease. Am J Otolaryngol 2009;30:337–9.
9. Zacharek MA, Fong KJ, Hwang PH. Image-guided frontal trephination: a minimally invasive approach for hard-to-reach frontal sinus disease. Otolaryngol Head Neck Surg 2006;135:518–22.
10. Jansen A. Neue Erfahrungen über chronische nebenhohleneiterungen der Nase. Arch Ohrennasen-Kehlkopfheilk 1902;56:110.
11. Ritter G. Eine neue Methode zur Erhaltung der vorderen Stirnhoehlenwand bei Radikaloperationen chronischer Stirnhoehleneiterungen. Dtsch Med Wochenschr 1906;32:1294–6.
12. Knapp. The Surgical Treatment of Orbital Complications in Diseases of the Nasal Accessory Sinuses. Journ Am Med Association 1908.
13. Lynch RC. The technique of a radical frontal sinus operation which has given me the best results. Laryngoscope 1921;31:1–5.
14. Howarth WG. Operations of the frontal sinus. J Laryngol Otol 1921;36:417–21.

15. Draf W. Endonasal frontal sinus drainage type I-III according to Draf. In: The frontal sinus. Germany: Springer Berlin Heidelberg; 2005. p. 219–32.
16. Yoon B-NA, Batra PS, Citardi MJ, et al. Frontal sinus inverted papilloma: surgical strategy based on the site of attachment. Am J Rhinol Allergy 2009;23:337–41.
17. Chiu AG, Schipor I, Cohen NA, et al. Surgical decisions in the management of frontal sinus osteomas. Am J Rhinol 2005;19(2):191–7.
18. Dedo HH, Broberg TG, Murr AH. Frontoethmoidectomy with Sewell-Boyden reconstruction: alive and well, a 25-year experience. Am J Rhinol 1998;12(3):191–8.
19. Amble FR, Kern EB, Neel B 3rd, et al. Nasofrontal duct reconstruction with silicone rubber sheeting for inflammatory frontal sinus disease: analysis of 164 cases. Laryngoscope 1996;106:809–15.
20. Benoit CM, Duncavage JA. Combined external and endoscopic frontal sinusotomy with stent placement: a retrospective review. Laryngoscope 2001;111(7):1246–9.
21. Rains BM 3rd. Frontal sinus stenting. Otolaryngol Clin North Am 2001;34(1):101–10.
22. Schonborn W. Ein beitrag zur casuistik der erkrankungen des sinus frontales. In: Wilkop A, editor. Wurzburg, Germany: F, Frome; 1894.
23. Brieger. Über chronische Eiterungen des nebenhohlen der Nase. Arch Ohren Nasen-Kehlkopfheilk 1895;39:213.
24. Marx H. Osteoma of the Nasal Accessory Sinuses with Rare Ocular Complications. Arch fur Ophthal 1910;74.
25. Hardy JM, Montgomery WW. Osteoplastic frontal sinusotomy: an analysis of 250 operations. Ann Otol Rhinol Laryngol 1976;85:523.
26. Bergara AR, Itoiz AO. Present state of the surgical treatment of chronic frontal sinusitis. Arch Otolaryngol 1955;61:616–28.
27. Tato JM, Sibbald DW, Bergaglis OE. Surgical treatment of the frontal sinus by the external route. Laryngoscope 1954;64:504–21.
28. Goodale RL, Montgomery WW. Experiences with the osteoplastic anterior wall approach to the frontal sinus. Arch Otolaryngol 1958;68:271–83.
29. Weber R, Draf W, Keerl R, et al. Osteoplastic frontal sinus surgery with fat obliteration: technique and long-term results using magnetic resonance imaging in 82 operations. Laryngoscope 2000;110(6):1037–44.
30. Courson AM, Stankiewicz JA, Lai D. Contemporary management of frontal sinus mucoceles: a meta-analysis. Laryngoscope 2014;124:378–86.

Index

Note: Page numbers of article titles are in **boldface** type.

Otolaryngol Clin N Am 49 (2016) 1091–1095
http://dx.doi.org/10.1016/S0030-6665(16)30097-4
0030-6665/16/$ – see front matter

oto.theclinics.com

Moving?

Make sure your subscription moves with you!

To notify us of your new address, find your **Clinics Account Number** (located on your mailing label above your name), and contact customer service at:

Email: journalscustomerservice-usa@elsevier.com

800-654-2452 (subscribers in the U.S. & Canada)
314-447-8871 (subscribers outside of the U.S. & Canada)

Fax number: 314-447-8029

Elsevier Health Sciences Division
Subscription Customer Service
3251 Riverport Lane
Maryland Heights, MO 63043

ELSEVIER

Printed and bound by CPI Group (UK) Ltd, Croydon, CR0 4YY

03/10/2024

01040395-0001